BRAIN
BODY
FOOD

——

Ngaire Hobbins

Author: **Ngaire Hobbins**

ABN: 25 699 506 380
Website: www.ngairehobbins.com
Facebook: www.facebook.com/ngairehobbinsdietitian
Instagram: ngairehobbins_dietitian
Twitter: @NgaireHobbins

ISBN: 978-0-6489145-0-9

CONTENTS

PREFACE

Thank you for picking up this book!

I wrote it for you who are interested in food, ageing and brain health. I am passionate about sharing my understanding of the current evidence on eating and living to enjoy the very best life into later years with everyday people and health professionals alike.

I am a clinically trained dietitian holding a Bachelor of Science degree with postgraduate qualifications in Nutrition and Dietetics. I am acknowledged as an authority in nutrition and ageing, and am a skilled presenter to groups of everyday people as well as professional audiences nationally and internationally.

The endless background chatter of self-proclaimed diet and nutrition gurus with little or no professional training in nutrition can make deciding what to eat from the tens of thousands of foods we encounter every day—many of which bear no resemblance to their healthy origins—challenging for those who just want to know how to live fulfilling, happy lives.

One of the wonderful benefits of significant life and career experience for me has been confirming what I always knew instinctively but is also increasingly supported by the weight of evidence—that my grandmother was doing most of the right things and fresh, minimally processed and, ideally, locally sourced food holds the answers to living well. About two decades ago I started working exclusively with older adults and discovered an almost complete lack of helpful, practical guidance specifically tailored to the needs of people enjoying unprecedented longevity.

Far too often in my clinical work over these years, I have seen physical and cognitive decline result from unawareness that nutrition needs beyond your mid 60s are not the same as they were in your younger years.

The blessings gained from longer lives also mean our bodies and brains need to endure the wear and tear of everyday life and continue to function for longer than they did in previous generations. Without a clear focus on the specific needs of living into these years, you become more vulnerable to infections, illnesses, wounds and falls and will struggle to recover from these. Fortunately, there is now a wealth of information available to help minimise the risk of physical and cognitive decline and to support these unique nutrition needs, so you can make the most of life as you grow old. My work is all about sharing that with you.

This book had its beginnings in my frustrations at seeing too many clients with physical and cognitive issues that could have been avoided had they understood the unique differences between the nutrition needs of their younger and older selves. I released *Eat To Cheat Ageing* in 2014 to counter the lack of good information and when the science of nutrition and brain health subsequently exploded, followed that in 2016 with *Eat To Cheat Dementia.* I have been asked many times to combine these books, so when an update was due I made the decision to do just that, merging the content into one manual for life into later age: *Brain, Body, Food* is the result.

Writing is somewhat of a necessary evil for me. It's my way to share knowledge with as many people as possible but is not a process I find comes easily and all that time spent in my head wrangling tens of thousands of words has wide ranging impacts on those around me. I fear that is most felt by my endlessly supportive and encouraging family—especially Craig and Jackson who again tolerated many months of a present-yet-absent wife and mother. I am so thankful to them and so many others: to my mother who believes I can achieve anything, to my regrettably more physically distant but equally adored and appreciated Nell, Angus, Anastasia and Mark, to Cathie, Penny, Vicki, Rosie, Anne-Marie, Ange, Robyn, Catherine and Sharee, the team at COTA Tasmania and my dad and Elaine who have patiently listened over and over to my frustrations and crazy ideas. To the wonderful Genevieve Lilley who let me be her very first 'writer in residence' in her glorious Cradle Mountain cottage. To my greatly loved and missed Avoca Beach book group and to the 'world's best geriatrician' Dr Peter Lipski, who together sent me on this path. And this book could never have come into existence without Rachael Bermingham's support, encouragement and excellent production coordination, all delivered with the perfect balance of fun, exuberance and professionalism.

Thank you all—this could never have happened had so many supports not been in place.

And may all who read this book enjoy fulfilling, joy-infused lives relishing every mouthful.

BODYWORKS

PART 1

Muscle: Your Anti-Ageing Frontline

*D*id you know the key to living a long and healthy life depends on more than merely avoiding illness? It lies in your muscles.

It's true. Muscles do a lot more than move you around—they hold the keys to you living the life you had hoped for in the years ahead. And they are more vulnerable than you might imagine.

You may have managed to keep up gym work, cycling, swimming or whatever is your thing, and secretly gloat over how athletic you look or maybe your muscles are now hidden by an extra bit of padding. No matter what's obvious on the surface or how you might feel, the unseen changes caused by inactivity, age, wear and tear, illness and stress can rob you of muscle minute by minute.

Why is that important?

Muscles do more for you than you may realise. They help maintain every one of your body's organs, help you avoid type 2 diabetes and ensure your brain is adequately fuelled to coordinate all your activity and keep your mind firing as you'd like it to. Muscles keep blood coursing in your veins to move oxygen, nutrients and fuel through your body. They also help you fight illness and infection and are essential for repair work, from everyday bumps and bruises to tissue, bone and tendon repair after major surgery.

Unfortunately, muscle loss is not always obvious until it has progressed far enough to have disastrous impact on physical and cognitive capacity, so being aware of its significance and working to head off any loss is essential. Medical advances may have managed to conquer illnesses that once claimed lives at a younger age, but making the most of the extra 20 years or so they have given us depends on finding ways to keep your body—especially your muscles—and brain going a lot longer than our grandparents might have needed to.

Generations ago eating meant hunting and gathering, and that meant running, climbing, throwing, digging, carrying really heavy stuff like whole animals, and walking, walking, walking. If you wanted to eat, you had no choice but to keep your muscles working. The hunter-gatherer lifestyle is no longer a career option and we have become far too good at finding ways to do less and less activity, which is bad news not only for our muscles but also for our immune system, our body organs and our brains. Nobody wants to return to the days of scrubbing floors on hands and knees, walking miles to work every day, or living without mod cons, but although these bygone lives seemed hard, they worked muscles as they needed to be worked.

My grandfather was born in the early 1900s. In those days 65 was considered a ripe old age—well and truly time to retire on the old age pension and potter around the house. Nowadays 65 is positively young! People expect far more from their remaining years than the generations before. We want to be able to travel, to get down and dirty with the grandkids, to embrace new technology—Skype, Facebook, perhaps online dating—and maybe take up belly dancing or skydiving.

Grandad had to chop and split wood and carry it up to the house every day just to get a cup of tea in the morning. He had to push a hand-mower across the lawn each Saturday; and if something had to be repaired, out came the hammer, the handsaw, the hand-drill and the manual screwdriver. Today we push a button to boil the jug, push a button to start the mower, which almost drives itself; and we can't imagine life without the electric drill, the chainsaw and perhaps even the electric nail gun.

Grandma did her washing in the copper, dragging each item out of scalding water with a stick and putting it through a hand wringer. If the sheets dared bunch up too much, the wringer had to be released, the washing unwound from the rollers, and the whole process started again. Then the very wet and heavy load had to be carried out to the washing line. The line was a floppy wire strung across the yard and propped up with long poles that needed to be angled low when Grandma pegged out the washing, then re-angled to hoist the washing higher to avoid dogs and small children playing in the washing as it dried (try doing that with a heavy load of wet washing on a line). She was judged by her good housekeeping and religiously mopped the floors and dragged the carpets bodily out of the house, draped them over the back fence, and beat the dust out of them with a cane carpet beater. She made cakes as light as air using only a wooden spoon, a hand-beater and elbow grease.

It's ironic: we've become so clever in thinking up endless arrays of gadgets and machines to do physical chores for us that we've outpaced the way our body systems have evolved. The fact is they still depend on us to keep them functioning well in order to continue to go about their work. I need to go to the gym to achieve the sort of strength and muscle Grandma took for granted.

The older you get, the more important muscles become.

It's fortunate that there is a lot you can do to keep your muscles up to scratch. Understanding what your muscles need is pivotal, and to do that you need to understand the role of what you eat. None of us want to give up our TV remotes, our washing machines or our electric drills, so we need to find alternative ways to keep the life in our muscles. That means not only staying active and doing exercise that boosts muscle, but also feeding them right, and that's about changing the focus from eating to avoid illness, to eating to age well.

Most health messages are aimed at the population as a whole and are often about avoiding the big baddies like heart disease. Those same messages need a different emphasis when you are looking to life ahead, beyond your late 60s. Of course it's still important to do what you can to avoid heart disease and other preventable illnesses—but living well into later age needs to be about more than preventing illness.

What you eat and do as you move beyond your 50s and 60s needs to be about tricking your body into thwarting what its physiology—the body's processing and functioning—naturally inclines it to do, which is to gradually slow down. Slowing down physiology-wise can mean your body systems not working as well as they once did. Thankfully though, while your muscles are affected by those system changes, they mainly slow down due to underuse but remain able to help you no matter your age, if you help them. Sure, illness can take a toll, but keeping your muscles working, and eating to support them is a pathway to heading off age-related physical and cognitive decline—giving you the power to make the most of the 20 or so years ahead.

To look more closely at how easily the wheels can fall off, consider Joan and Betty:

Joan and Betty did most things together. There was golf, a bit of tennis, plenty of socialising and getting out and about with friends and families. Joan was always just a bit more active and always seemed able to eat yet stay thin, while Betty struggled to keep her weight down most of her life. Both slowed down a bit from their mid 50s, but not enough to cause any concern. Life was good and they felt they'd earned a chance to rest up a bit.

However, as Joan did less she also found herself feeling less hungry, and her meals became smaller. She was conscious of maintaining her health and read up on various diets. Her daughter had recently had success with one where she ate mostly fruit, salads, vegetables and wholegrain foods, with just occasional meats and fish and some low fat dairy foods, so Joan took that on. Her friend Betty just enjoyed her food too much to cut down. She tried to share her friend's interest in her diet and managed to go along with it some of the time, though not always with the same determination or success.

When Joan lost some weight she wasn't worried. She felt quite virtuous. Betty didn't lose any but didn't gain either, so felt she was doing okay. By 68 they both felt well and were living good, healthy lives.

This all seems perfectly reasonable and appropriately healthy, right? Wrong!

There are some red flags in this picture that may surprise you. They are weight loss, eating smaller meals, and eating fewer high-protein foods. Joan was well intentioned, but while the diet she chose was great for her 43-year-old daughter, it was not the best for her.

Age imposes unique nutritional needs, no matter how well you eat or what you weigh. What Joan and Betty didn't know is that losing weight when you are older means losing muscle, and that sets you up for poor health ahead. Those smaller meals Joan had been choosing along with less meat and dairy, meant getting fewer essentials, like protein.

Now is the time to review and realign your ideal food choices, even for those of you like Betty, who felt so far from Joan's lack of interest in food and her ability to gradually lose weight that she might as well have inhabited another planet. Of the two, Betty was actually better off when it came to staying independent and healthy into the future.

That 'healthy' diet you might have been trying hard to stick with may no longer be right for you.

We'll come back to the girls soon—let's look in more detail at the hidden benefits of body muscle.

Figure 1:

Body muscle helps you in more ways than you might expect. It:

> Supports your immune system so you can fight infection and illness

> Supports repair of wounds and recovery from illness

> Helps you to continue to swallow safely and effectively

> Helps maintain a healthy appetite

> Helps your body use its insulin effectively to avoid diabetes developing or its symptoms worsening

> Helps keep fuel supplied to your brain

> Helps you avoid having an adverse reaction to a medication

> Stops you from falling should you lose balance or miss your step

> Allows you to keep moving around engaging in physical activity

> Supports your joints to reduce the pain of arthritis and maintain flexibility.

WHY MUSCLE IS MORE TO YOU THAN MERELY WHAT MOVES YOU

Your muscles are your reserve supply of body protein.

Why is that important? Because protein is constantly being used to fight illness and infection, do the body's repair work, keep body organs functioning and help support brain fuel supply.

Every little thing your body has to do every minute of every day means wear and tear on your cells. And every cell in every organ—in your skin, your gut, your blood, as well as all the substances running the systems that keep you alive—has a lifespan. Some have only hours of life, some days, some months before they are replaced. Protein is used minute by minute to address wear and tear, to repair damage and for constant renewal. At the same time it's helping fight off infection and fuelling your brain—as we'll see later on.

I eat food, and food contains protein, so what's the problem?

It's more about continuity of supply: we don't eat 24 hours a day, but protein is needed all that time. That's where the muscle protein reserve comes in.

It's rather like your car. Once you turn that key, you expect to be able to travel a long way. Your car needs fuel to keep running but you don't carry the petrol station or the power source around with you for that constant supply. Your car's fuel tank or battery is your reserve between fill-ups; and muscle is our protein reserve between food fill-ups. Unlike your car, which you can switch off when its work is done, the demand for protein doesn't stop, even when you are sleeping or relaxing on the couch, and there are always going to be gaps between protein coming in from food.

Protein is released from your muscles to bridge those gaps, which come along surprisingly often: they include the non-eating hours between meals; the times when you are unwell and just can't eat properly; or if you fast—for medical, religious or other reasons. And there are always days when you just don't get time to eat the meals you should.

In a car you start with a full tank, travelling along at whatever pace you choose. If you don't refuel, a time will come when you will just stop. It's different for your body—it's not all or nothing. If your protein reserve dwindles enough, all the systems that rely on it start to falter and you face more of a series of steps down towards a slow, grinding halt.

Fortunately, even those of us who don't look like Mr or Ms

Universe are blessed with a start-up muscle supply that is built as we grow to peak adulthood. That supply can easily keep us cruising along until about our mid 60s. And let's face it, anyone now in their later years understands that not long ago, 70 was positively old!

Nowadays the extra two or three decades mean muscles need some help if they're going to be that protein reserve: to keep you moving, but also to help you fight illness and infection, repair injuries, keep your body organs running, avoid type 2 diabetes (or manage it if you already have it) and more.

Holding onto the muscle you have, boosting it if needed and replenishing it as much as possible will always keep plenty of protein in reserve for when you need it.

Back to Joan and Betty:

Around comes the cold and flu season and Joan succumbs. You know what it's like with the flu—you don't always feel like eating. Joan's muscle reserve starts furiously releasing protein to augment what little food she is able to eat. Her immune system is able to rage along on the protein reserves supplied by her muscles while food isn't available to do the job, and Joan recovers.

Betty and other friends are shocked when they see her next— she has clearly lost weight. Joan is not as concerned. She thinks weight loss is always good.

She is mistaken, a lot of the kilograms she has lost will be muscle (read more about this soon), which has the potential to cause her more harm than good, even if she has lost some body fat.

For things to reset to how they were before her illness, Joan needs to replace the muscle (and protein reserve) she has lost, not to mention the weight loss prior to that. Betty would be in a better position, not having already lost weight. It's Joan who is the concern—and this is where age raises its somewhat unattractive head: the older you get the harder it is to rebuild muscle. Not just because exercise becomes less appealing, but also because of the age bias of our physiology.

WE ARE PHYSIOLOGICALLY DRIVEN TO GROW THAT ADULT BODY, BUT NOT TO GET BIGGER ONCE WE GET THERE

Humans are beautifully designed with systems, which use the food we eat and oxygen we breathe from our first moment on earth to build the body we achieve at peak adulthood—around our mid 40s. However, if that growth continued, we would all be giants by 60! That's clearly not the case: things change.

On the way to your peak, the more you use your muscles, the more they build and support your health in a myriad of ways; even without doing much muscle work, you are hard wired to grow and build them. And if any get lost because your muscle reserve is needed temporarily to provide protein for rescue work, this convenient programming drives rebuilding as soon as you eat again.

That programmed rebuilding relies on a combination of three things:

1. Messages from hormones

2. Signals from nerves

3. The activity of the muscles themselves.

And here's where our bodies' ageist physiology strikes against us. Hormone levels diminish and the signals from nerves dwindle with age. From as early as your 30s or 40s both are affected, and by your mid 60s the hormone and nerve boosting of muscles that built you up to your peak structure, has all but ceased.

That leaves muscle activity alone in the rebuilding task—but your muscles are reminded to repair and build only when you work them. Fortunately, even though it gets more difficult to completely rebuild the older you get, that system does keep working as long as you live.

So, if your body is to have any chance at all of keeping pace with the plans you've made for the years ahead, it needs your help. Those flabby arms and bingo wings, flibberty bits, saggy bottoms and turkey necks may be gravity's joke, but under that exterior it's up to you to nurture your inner Adonis. That means considering five things:

1. Eating for your muscles: protein, protein, protein.

Ironically, after all those years when most of us seemed to struggle to keep our meal sizes within civilised boundaries, when we were often being told to eat less meat and dairy and that the pinnacle of good nutrition was a plate piled to the ceiling with salad and veggies topped with nothing but a squeeze of lemon, the time has now come for a lot of that to be turned on its head. Not everyone is going to find they eat less food as they get older, but improbable as it seems, many of us will. And while all those lovely vegetables, fruits and leafy things provide irreplaceable vitamin and antioxidant boosters, the meats, cheeses and nuts of this world take on an elevated status from now on.

Why? Because you are still running an adult-sized body no matter how old you are, and it still has adult-sized needs for most nutrients. In fact, with all the extra wear and tear that occurs as you age, you need more of some things than you did when you were younger, and protein is one of them. So the importance of packing extra nutrition into your meals to keep your muscles up to scratch and cheat ageing is undeniable. You don't have to eat huge amounts of protein foods, but you mustn't eat less than you did when younger.

People over 70 are thought to need at least 20% more protein than in younger years. Figure 2 gives you a basic guide to protein foods, with much more detail provided later in Foodworks.

Figure 2:

FOODS SUPPLYING PROTEIN	
All meats, poultry, offal, fish, seafoods:	focus mainly on fresh cuts, enjoying processed varieties like ham, bacon and smoked meats/seafoods less frequently
Eggs:	chicken or any other
Dairy foods:	including liquid, concentrated (evaporated) and dried milk, cheese and yoghurt (but not cream or butter, which like oils, are not high protein) milk, cheese, yoghurt from goats, sheep or other
Soy products:	including soy beverages, yoghurt, tofu, tempeh and others
Pulses:	including baked beans, peas, broad beans, lentils, chickpeas, kidney and similar beans

Nuts, seeds:	all varieties (whole or ground) and products made from them (apart from their oils, which do not contain protein)
Hemp products:	including seeds, hulled seeds and flour (apart from hemp oil, which has no protein)
High-protein powdered supplements:	including skim milk powder, whey protein isolate products plant-based isolates and powders from soy, peas, hemp rice and others.

Life is too short to spend thinking about every mouthful you take, so make it easy for yourself: put a good protein food at the centre of every meal and you won't have to struggle to keep up the supply.

When you ate larger meals, you could easily get away with only having protein foods at some meals or in very small amounts as a 'garnish' while vegetables, fruits and grains held centre stage. In fact, that's the ideal diet plan to combat obesity in younger people, and you might believe it is right for older adults from reading, watching or listening to eating advice in the popular press, online or even from medical or public health authorities.

However, so much of that generalist advice fails to take into account the unique needs of older adults: unless you include a good protein food at most meals you risk not being able to cope with your body's demands. If you do suffer an illness or an infection you will need to eat more protein to help balance what your muscles will lose so you can repair and recover, but be aware this might mean eating extra protein between meals and for some, high protein drinks or supplements might be necessary. There is more detailed guidance on protein in foods and how to plan to get what you need in Foodworks.

2: Does it matter where the protein comes from: animal versus vegetable?

It doesn't matter to your body where the protein in your meals comes from. Because you probably aren't eating as much as you did when you were younger, you need to pack more protein and other essentials into every serve or every mouthful.

Many animal-based foods have an advantage because servings of meat, fish or dairy don't always need to be as large to give the same amount of protein as they usually do when the protein comes from plant-based foods (such as soy milk, nuts, seeds or grains). The amount of protein in foods does vary as you can see in figure 3, so it is important if you prefer to eat fewer animal-based protein foods that the plant foods you choose give you the protein you need. Head to Foodworks for more on protein in foods and practical strategies to get what you need from your meals and snacks.

Figure 3:

Animal vs vegetable: comparison of approximate cooked serve sizes to get an equivalent amount (20g) of protein	
Cheese (cheddar)	40g – about half cup grated or matchbox-sized piece
Meat, chicken, fish	60g – meat portion (about size of 1 pack of cards)/ 1 lge chicken drumstick/ 2/3 small can tuna/salmon drained
Eggs	150g – 3 X 50g eggs

Tofu	140g – portion about size of 2 packs of cards
Lentils/chick peas	220g – a generous cup or half a can
Nuts/LSA mix	200g – about 1 cup
Mushrooms (fresh)	450g – enough to half fill a bucket
Rice/quinoa	660g – about 6 cups

Researchers in sports science and in space programs have looked at which proteins work best in building muscle. For athletes it's obviously vital to tailor muscle bulk and strength for peak performance. For astronauts, the absence of gravity removes a lot of the drive to maintain and build muscle that occurs when we just move about on earth and can have devastating consequences if not well managed. It's ridiculously expensive to provide exercise for astronauts during space travel so the food they are provided must help their muscles to get the most from the time they can exercise.

Researchers have found that the animal proteins they tested helped build more muscle than the plant proteins. Not every protein known to man has been tested but it seems the benefit is a consequence of the amino acids they contain. Of 20 amino acids humans use, most are interchangeable to build whichever protein is needed in the body or brain, but some are 'essential', meaning we must get them from the food we eat—no substitution is possible. Of those found in human muscle, leucine seems to be especially important. Proteins with higher leucine content seem to be useful for muscle building when they are eaten close to the time you exercise (ideally within an hour).

There is a list of some foods and their leucine contents in Foodworks.

Building and maintaining muscle is of immense importance to athletes, but even if you are not planning to run a four-minute mile any day soon, your muscles will benefit in the same way.

What about animal protein foods and cholesterol?

Years ago, concerns about fat and cholesterol may have had you eating less meat, eggs and dairy; but those concerns don't stack up quite the same way at a later age. Protein is now much more important, and the other nutrients those foods supply are a bonus. Low fat diets are no longer what most need.

As you read on you will understand more and more about why it's time to ditch some of the concerns of your youth and enjoy one of the benefits of reaching a mature age.

3: Providing memory jogs to those forgetful muscles

Like you and me, muscles like to be reminded they're needed. There's no getting around the saying, 'use it or lose it'. Sure, it's harder to keep your muscles the way they were, but unless you keep using them, and using them well, they'll forget what they're there for.

That means you need to think about the type of muscle activity you do. First of all, there's the benefit of gravity. Our muscles thrive on the effects of gravity and you can use that to your advantage by avoiding sitting or lying down too much. Of course you need to rest, but don't get complacent: keep looking for ways that gravity can help you every day: get up, stand tall, move around, carry things, use the stairs, park farther from the shop, walk instead of drive, rake the lawn, sweep the floor. There are endless examples. If you happen to enjoy some water-based activity, the action of moving against the water in swimming or aqua aerobics classes also gives your muscles a good reminder, without the impact of gravity.

Then there is exercise itself. Sadly, it's just not enough any more to stroll around the shops or go for a leisurely walk. In order to boost muscle function at every chance, you need to do activities that stress your muscles and help make up for those absent hormones and vastly diminished nerve triggers. And because you have muscles everywhere, it has to be an activity that works not only your legs, but also your upper body, arms and abdomen. Your muscles need to work against a weight (resistance exercise) to encourage them to build.

Luckily, 'resistance' doesn't have to mean lifting weights in a gym. Walking briskly or uphill, swimming laps or doing aqua aerobics, sweeping or raking the leaves, taking the stairs more often, even doing supervised exercises like tai chi or over 50s fitness classes are all good, as long as they get your heart rate up and have you puffing and sweating a little. See below for a list of suggested activities to maintain your muscles.

All these activities need to be checked with your doctor first and carefully supervised as you get older, but that doesn't mean you shouldn't do them. Using age as a reason to do less physical activity, to sit most of the day and have daytime naps, will only do harm in the long run.

As soon as possible after being immobilised or bed ridden due to illness, accident or any other reason, you must work extra hard to help recover any muscle that's been lost. It may not be what you feel like doing, but immobilisation removes those essential muscle reminders and mustn't be ignored if you want to return to the activities you enjoy, or you could face ongoing illness and declining health.

> *Joan and Betty were wrong to believe that what Joan had read in magazines and diet books applied to them, and they were wrong to believe that slowing down and eating less was 'just a part of getting older'.*

The rules about what is good for you now you are older are not the same as when you were younger. If you could count on living only until your late 60s, your muscle reserves might well hold out without much help. However, as you are likely to live well past that age, your health and independence in the future depend on your muscle reserves still being there when you need them in your 80s and beyond. And that won't happen without you making the effort.

Figure 4: Guidelines for exercise to help maintain muscle function

The ideal is to combine aerobic, resistance, flexibility and balance activities, so you need to find activities you are able to do that don't put you at risk of falling; and ideally that interest you. Professional assistance is ideal but not essential. Everyday activities like vacuuming and mopping, raking, sweeping, gardening, carrying the shopping and doing housework contribute, but adopting the following are your best bet to cheat ageing:

Aerobic

> › On at least 3 days per week initially, increasing to every day

> Aim for 30 to 60 minutes each day, which can be accumulated in 10 minute bouts

> Make at least 20 or 30 minutes of this time at vigorous intensity (puffing and sweating).

Resistance

> Weight training at least 2 days per week

> Do exercises for all major muscle groups: legs, arms, abdomen, hips, back, chest, shoulders

> Use a weight you can just manage for 8–10 repetitions for each muscle group, and when it gets easy to do more than that, increase the weight (more effective than doing extra repetitions).

Flexibility

> Do sustained stretches for each major muscle group on at least 2 days a week

> Use static stretches, don't 'bounce' or use movement during stretches.

Balance

> On at least 1 day a week, working up to every day, do 4 to 10 different balance activities in a safe environment, repeating each 1or 2 times.

Figure 5: Exercise guidelines for recovery after illness or immobilisation

Resistance exercise is the most important for recovery. Don't expect it to increase the size of your muscles as that's unlikely, but it will help in your recovery, boost your strength and ability, and improve your longer-term health. You can start with either no weights or very light ones, but add extra when you can, or do extra repetitions on the same weight so you progress in strength.

As soon as you are able—even while you are confined to bed (and as long as it's safe to do so)—start to do as much as you can even if it's only one or two activities at first. Work up to doing 8 to 12 repetitions of exercises for each major muscle group: legs, arms, abdomen, hips, back, chest, shoulders.

If you have had surgery or an injury and are in hospital, check what you are able to do with the physiotherapist or ask your doctor.

As soon as you are able to, return to doing all your maintenance activities.

4: The damage done by bed rest: it's like being in outer space for your muscles.

Being immobilised by illness—also somewhat misleadingly called 'bed rest'—is more harmful to your muscles than merely leading an inactive life. It affects your body much the same way as being in zero gravity does an astronaut, and it's worse the older you get. It actively robs you of muscle, which doesn't come back automatically when you are older.

If you have had an accident, surgery or sickness, chances are you will spend some time in bed, and during that time your muscles won't get their usual workout. That includes the everyday fight against gravity to keep you upright as well as everything else you do to remind your muscles what they are there for. So, although you may not feel like doing anything more active than eating delightful hospital cuisine and drinking insipid tea while confined to bed, you are going to lose muscle if you don't get up and do some exercise as soon as you can.

There is a little bit of a silver lining: some of the lost muscle becomes protein reserve and is diverted into repairing wounds, combating infection or fighting off fever. Unfortunately, the combined loss through diversion into repair work and lack of exercise can be large. Realising what's going on and working to minimise the effects can be your key to stopping a vicious cycle of muscle loss and illness, which could trigger increasing frailty and chronic ill health. Get active as soon as you are able, so that muscle loss won't become permanent.

To be clear, you might also lose body fat with this type of weight loss, but that's not the bonus you think it is because weight loss during immobilisation, illness or after surgery is a sign that all-important muscle has also certainly been lost.

If the time in bed is only a day or two it might seem like there's little to be worried about: it might be unavoidable and you need to enjoy the rest. Research with healthy individuals has shown that 10 days in bed can easily rob you of 1kg of muscle and that is a lot to lose. If you are very unwell (during a serious illness like pneumonia, a major surgery or a pressure injury) that same amount can be lost in just four days and losses will continue as long as you remain immobile. (*see* **figure 6** *on muscle loss impacts below*)

This is the time for getting good protein and doing everything you can to move as soon as you possibly can. If that's not possible then you must move on to good rehabilitation including exercise and eating that builds muscle.

Daytime rests can also be an issue if they get out of hand. A 'nanna nap', or the '40 winks' often mentioned in my family, can certainly be replenishing, but too much rest time every day just means your muscles are missing out.

Figure 6: How much muscle do I have and how can losing it affect me?

> **The amount of muscle we have varies enormously depending on our genetics and how much resistance exercise we do regularly. For most moderately active people in the healthy weight range, muscle is usually about 40% of bodyweight.**
>
> > ❯ Muscle loss increases your chance of gaining excess weight and your likelihood of developing type 2 diabetes or hampering management if you already have diabetes
> >
> > ❯ During a major illness, losing just 5% of body muscle reduces the function of your internal organs and slows wound healing
> >
> > ❯ With a loss of around 20% body muscle, organs begin to fail
> >
> > ❯ Death can result from a 40% body muscle loss.

5: The problem of an over-enthusiastic immune system.

Your immune system is able to rally the 'protein troops' to mount a defence almost the instant a foreign substance enters your body. It's working before you're even aware you've been invaded, and it can neutralise a threat before any symptoms get the chance to appear.

It's an awesome response plan and it efficiently protects you from illness. Specialised immune substances are made from protein as soon as the system starts up and that continues as long as there is a need. That protein can come from your last meal, but between meals and anytime you are not eating well, it's muscle protein that is used.

A strong immune system requires balance: too much immune activity can be as damaging as too little. Part of the immune response depends on inflammation, which is important in rallying the body's defences, but it's also where too much activity can cause problems. The condition known as chronic inflammation (or what is often known as CLIP—chronic low-grade inflammatory profile—in medical terms) is covered in more detail in Brainworks but needs mention here.

At a later age, the immune system can be slow to switch off after an illness—remaining active longer than is necessary and contributing to chronic inflammation. As a result small amounts of muscle can continue to be lost even when you have recovered or are feeling quite well—often for long periods of time. Sometimes your immune system can react when there is no real threat, and that's a big problem for your muscles because targeting unwanted invaders, whether real or not uses muscle protein.

You won't always know that muscle has been lost, although weight loss may be a tell-tale sign. When you are older, you should always assume that you have to actively rebuild your muscle reserves after any illness. The same recovery strategies you put in place after immobilisation will also help head off any lingering losses after illness.

The gut microbiome: protection and impacts on immune response.

You may have read about the amazing influence the billions of bacteria living inside your gastrointestinal tract (or more simply, your gut) have on your mood, behaviour and the health of your brain and that is discussed in detail in Brainworks.

What I'd like to touch on here is the protective role of the gut microbiome. While anything we put in our mouths contains an array of things that are good for us, there are always going to be some that can do us harm. The gut microbiome monitors what's there, 'senses' those that are bad and passes the information on to the gut–brain axis, from where an immune response is coordinated.

That response tends to have two stages: vomiting and diarrhoea is the first line of defence, causing a rapid removal of the offending contents. The second line of defence gets a bit more complex. The brain and the gut bacteria influence the 'leakiness' of the gut wall as well as transit time. The leakiness determines what substances can easily get from the gut into the blood and the transit time is how fast the gut contents are moved along from mouth to anus.

These changes can be powerful over time in much the same way as an over-reactive immune system: excessive leakiness allows substances that usually can't get through the gut wall to do so, which can potentially cause problems. In contrast, if the gut contents are pushed through too quickly, there is not enough time for all the valuable nutrients to be absorbed.

When something that shouldn't slips through the gut wall, the second line of defence swings into action with an impressive array of resources including a number of substances that trigger inflammation.

You now know inflammation is an important part of the immune response and that it must be controlled. The problem with the leaky gut is that it can trigger autoimmune problems and chronic inflammation, and because the gut–brain axis is in play, emotions and anxiety can also be influenced.

There is a lot going on and we have much more to learn about the gut–brain axis, but we know that increased diversity in the microbiome and 'good' bacteria tend to help reduce excessive leakiness and dampen over-inflammation as well as have the potential to positively influence emotion, anxiety, mood and more. In contrast, the opposite is true of reduced diversity and a higher proportion of 'bad' bacteria.

How did Joan and Betty go, you ask?

Well, in true happy-ending tradition, they got great advice, both revved up their activity levels, started to eat more good-protein foods, and felt so much better that they took up pole dancing at 70! (Well, no, that's just a rumour—as far as we know—but they did go on a cruise, and kicked up their heels!)

It's easy, and mostly common sense, to avoid muscle loss setting you up for ill health, but many people inadvertently make lifestyle choices that don't help them. Muscle can be lost for many years before stick-thin arms and legs make it physically obvious, and all the while the body's systems, which rely on that muscle protein reserve, can be faltering. It's hard to reverse if it goes on too long; avoidance is so much easier.

BODYWORKS

PART 2

A 'Wicked Problem': The Need to Consider Bodyweight Differently at Later Age.

*H*ere's when being older is suddenly the best thing. The quick answer at least to the boring old question about what you should weigh is, 'Whatever you weigh now—don't go losing any!'

Being told that *avoiding* losing weight is the best thing for you now might not be the impression you get from the latest diets in glossy magazines, from what's being blasted at you by your TV, on the web, or even the advice of some doctors, dietitians and self-appointed health gurus. That's pretty much because all that advice is for the youngsters out there. It might be great advice for 30-, 40- or 50-year-olds, but you can finally ignore the endless 'diet to lose weight NOW' mantra.

The science is clear: once you are in your late 60s or beyond, weight loss diets are not good news.

That's because, from now on, losing weight by dieting—no matter how good the diet sounds—means losing muscle; and while that might not be obvious, either in your everyday activities or in how you look, we now know that it sets you up for ill health and squanders your independence. Sure, if you lose weight, some of that may be fat—but since muscle will always have gone along with that, it's not a plus in the end.

It is possible to lose weight without losing too much muscle at a later age, but it requires the right exercise and many people leave that part out, or don't do enough, convinced that the latest diet trend is adequate. There is no alternative to moving and pushing your muscles.

It might take a magic mirror to reflect the Venus or Adonis you know is inside you when your gym body seems to be have been mysteriously replaced by a wax replica that looks as if it has been left out in the sun, but every bit of muscle in your body under the surface is adding life to your years.

I often see older people who have lost four or five kilos (8 or 10lb) without any conscious effort, and that's not good news. The muscle reduction as a result of that weight loss can already be affecting their health without them even being aware of it.

I know that for those of you who have always been a bit fatter than you 'should be' and struggled for years to keep your weight down, this is a mix of bitter and sweet: bitter because if you find you've lost weight you are going to feel virtuous, even smug, and then along comes an annoying dietitian saying you shouldn't have! It's also sweet, because finally it's okay to not be 'on a diet'.

Surely obesity is bad for my health!

Yes, it is.

Don't for one minute imagine that being obese or overweight in younger people is good—it's not! In fact, being significantly overweight in your early 60s, 50s or younger is associated with inflammation in the body and brain and you are at higher risk of dementia as well as other obesity-related illnesses.

Something researchers are looking at is whether obesity in early and middle adulthood contributes to 'leakiness' in the blood brain barrier. It seems it might and if so, it makes the brain vulnerable to substances that shouldn't be able to pass that protective barrier. This is covered in more detail in Brainworks.

The grim truth is that too many people who have been inactive and obese through their younger lives don't actually make it into their late 80s for all sorts of reasons.

There is so much research going on in this area, but the advice that results is no different to the rest of this book—avoid excessive weight in early and middle adulthood and stay active throughout life—it's never too late to boost muscle.

The time to lose excess weight is well before your late 60s. From then on, if you are very overweight it's really too late to safely do anything about it by yourself.

If the excess kilos you carry have brought on, or are worsening, your diabetes; if they make getting around harder; or worsen joint, arthritic or other issues, then carrying less weight would of course make life easier and reduce your chances of further health problems. Even so, trying to do anything about your weight just by dieting will do more harm than good; you must also exercise to head off muscle loss. Any exercise you can do yourself is great (a thorough medical examination before you begin anything new is highly advisable), but only a good exercise program that includes resistance activity can help you avoid muscle loss if you take up any sort of diet designed to shed kilos or pounds.

The exercises previously outlined in **figure 4** to maintain and boost muscle will give you a guide, but it would be best to follow a structured program designed specifically for what you need and what you are able to do, and you must commit yourself to continuing with it from now on.

The way you live your life has a long term effect: a sedentary lifestyle, particularly the proportion of time spent sitting compared to moving around is a strong driver of obesity. Relaxation is good for the soul, and some down time is important in day-to-day life, but the balance has been thrown out of kilter by our modern lifestyles.

If you are now in your late 70s or beyond, you are at a decided advantage because you grew up when life was less sedentary. You cannot afford to become complacent now, but anyone younger especially needs to take heed. There is far too much inactive time available to us and many of us have become far too used to enjoying it. Every minute you are inactive reduces the time you are up and about, burning kilojoules and boosting muscle. No matter what you weigh, if you spend less time watching TV, sitting at the computer or in an armchair, driving in the car or sitting on a bus, and more time walking, standing, gardening, or doing any sort of physical activity you will help your body and your brain, even if it doesn't strip off kilos.

Ruth's story

Ruth had been a large lady since having her children. She was not an active person and had suffered a number of health and mobility problems since her late 50s.

She moved into a hostel in her late 60s when she needed a

bit more help and wasn't able to get on the bus as well as she had. By her late 70s, her mobility was quite reduced and the nursing supervisor in the hostel suggested she should see a dietitian to help her lose weight.

I was asked to see Ruth.

She was a lovely, friendly lady. On the BMI chart she was certainly in the weight category of very-overweight-to-obese. She had good friends in the hostel and they did all the bus trips and went out for coffee at least two or three times a week, even though she was wheelchair-bound most of the day. She kept a supply of sweets and other treats in her room 'for the grandkids' and to 'share with the nurses'. Ruth's diet was, in fact, quite good. She was not eating extreme amounts of kilojoules and had not gained any weight for years. Certainly, she would have been better able to get around if she was lighter, and it was understandable that the nurses thought it a good idea for her to lose weight. But she wasn't able to do the exercise needed to maintain her muscle through weight loss. Changing her diet so she lost weight would have been harmful to Ruth and put her at higher risk of illness, not to mention restricting some foods that brought joy to her life.

The hostel had access to a physiotherapist so we were able to discuss possible exercise options for Ruth and she was able to start on some very gentle workouts, however they really weren't enough to achieve much muscle building, if any.

Here was a lady who, at nearly 80, enjoyed her meals, and whose main source of pleasure in life revolved around the treats she shared with her grandchildren and her friends at their coffee sessions. Looking at the bigger picture, it was not going to be possible to get Ruth to lose weight by dieting without potentially harming her health through loss of muscle. Not to mention that Ruth was not keen on the idea and it was likely to reduce the enjoyment she gained from life. The advice to the facility had to be that weight loss was not advisable for Ruth at her age.

It was a very different picture for Margaret.

Margaret's story

Margaret was a lady in her mid 70s who was very overweight, had been for years, and was starting to struggle to get around as well as she would have liked. She had been diagnosed with type 2 diabetes in the last year and was taking medication for high blood pressure. Margaret was advised to attend a local gym program especially designed for seniors, and she started on a program of exercises and activities to strengthen her muscles and increase her exercise capacity. While she found it very hard at first, the boost to her energy levels and improvement in her ability to do everything from carrying the shopping, to pushing her grandkids in the stroller made it worth the effort, and after a short while she began to enjoy her sessions. She felt she was enjoying the rest of life more, and, much to her relief, was able to reduce her blood pressure medication and even avoid taking medication for her diabetes. Her diet wasn't restricted as part of her training, but she was assisted by the dietitian to plan meals and snacks with plenty of different foods, making sure she got the protein she needed. The treats she was fond of were not forbidden, but she did find she was eating fewer of them as she varied her meals more and felt better.

Her weight didn't change much but she was stronger and healthier, and felt far happier.

Exercise is not completely out of reach, no matter how overweight or how frail you may be. What is important is planning activities that are medically and physically appropriate.

What about the link between being overweight and type 2 diabetes? Shouldn't I be worried?

Type 2 diabetes is a major health issue, but in older age especially, lack of exercise plays a bigger role than being overweight. When muscle is active it helps your body use insulin efficiently and supports the activity of your diabetes medications. If you are inactive or immobile, the help your muscles can provide is reduced and your diabetes can worsen.

Certainly, excess weight in younger age is a major player in the development of diabetes, so if you are still in your 60s or younger it's especially important to act right away to reduce your chances of diabetes developing or worsening. Activity and exercise—involving both aerobic and resistance strategies—will improve your diabetes control whether you lose weight in the process or not.

Diabetes is covered in greater detail in Healthworks. Here it's sufficient to say that the same rule applies to people with or without diabetes: that is, do everything you can to boost your muscles and don't aim to lose weight by dieting alone.

Being a bit overweight is better for your health than being very lean now.

It's true. The science is quite clear: people now over 65 who are a bit heavier have fewer health problems and are likely to live longer than those who are very thin.

There are all sorts of guides for you to check where your weight, waist measurement and body fat fit so you can feel virtuous or devastated, depending on the outcome. The BMI (Body Mass Index) is not ideal for older people but is well known and is quite easy to use so it's often discussed. The 'healthy weight range' it identifies (BMI between 20 and 24) doesn't clearly distinguish between young and old. It really applies best to people not yet in their 70s.

The healthy weight range—whichever way you measure and compare it—is not about fashion: it's about the body weight that gives you the best chance of good health and longer life. Exactly what this is, and how it applies to people moving into later years is an area that has been under intense discussion among scientists and health authorities in the past few years. Among advisory groups and health professionals working specifically with older people, there is general agreement that the BMI for older adults should advise a lower level of 22. The upper range varies between groups but commonly is 27. A healthy weight range of 22-27 for those 70+ means that what just a few years ago might have labelled you as overweight (for example a BMI of 26) is now recognised as being healthy, while a BMI of 21, which would have been regarded as ideal for the younger you, now finds you too thin.

There have been many research studies that have found people with a BMI around 30 (in the obese range for younger adults) faring better than those with a BMI below 22.

If this seems strange to you, read on. It's partly about muscles again because muscle is heavier than body fat; so if you lead an active life and are doing regular exercise you could also have a higher BMI than someone less active. And in that case, because being more active is absolutely ideal for your health, so too is the higher BMI.

What's also possible is that heavier people are eating more food and thus getting more protein and anti-ageing nutrients to help them. Or that having to carry a bit of extra weight makes their muscles and bones work harder—also a good thing for keeping them going.

It could also be that fat actually does something other than just boost cuddliness. Body fat cells produce small amounts of hormones that might help protect brain function once you are older, and when body fat is lost, so is that protection.

Whatever the reasons, the message remains: overweight in early and middle age is a problem, but after your late 60s, it is no longer appropriate to consider dieting to lose weight, and being a bit cuddly is no longer a bad thing—in fact it's probably good for you.

Figure 7: Science shows it's healthier to carry a little extra weight when you are older

Scientific studies of large numbers of older people over recent years found:

> People already 70 to 75 years of age were 13% more likely to die in the following five years if they had a BMI in the 19 to 25 range, than if they had a BMI of 25 to 30 (the former is usually considered 'normal weight' for younger adults and the latter 'overweight')

> Older women with a BMI below 22. 5 and men below 23 (both classified in the mid range of 'normal' weight for younger adults) have more chance of experiencing ill health or dying compared to those with a BMI between 23 and 28.2

> Nursing home residents, even those with a BMI that would put them in the obese range at a younger age (a BMI of more than 30), fare better health-wise than those who have a lower BMI

> In a study of people aged 70 to 75 in Europe, the BMI at which people were least likely to die from any cause in the following 10 years was 27, a level considered overweight among younger adults

> Irrespective of starting weight, in post-menopausal women an unintentional loss of as little as 5% of body weight in one year (that's only 3kg (7lb) if you weigh 60kg (132lb), or 3.5kg if you are 70kg) is associated with increased risk of death in 5 to 10 years. It's likely to be similar for men

> If elderly people are very lean they suffer more complications in surgery than heavier people.

[1] Flicker, L., et al. 2010 'Body mass index and survival in men and women aged 70 and 75', Journal of the American Geriatric Association 58 (2); 234-241

[2] Price, GM., et al. 2006 'Weight, shape and mortality risk in older persons: elevated waist-hip ratio, not high body mass index, is associated with a greater risk of death', American Journal of Clinical Nutrition 84; 449-460

[3] Bahat, G., et al. 2102 'Which body mass index (BMI) is better in the elderly for functional status?', Archives of Gerontology and Geriatrics 54 (1); 78-81

[4] DeHollander, EL., et al. 2012 'The impact of body mass index in old age on cause-specific mortality', Journal of Nutrition, Health and Ageing 16 (1); 100-106

[5] Diehr, P., et al. 2008 'Weight, mortality, years of healthy life and active life expectancy in older adults', Journal of the American Geriatrics Society 56; 76-83

[6] Miller, SL. & Wolfe, RR. 2008 'The danger of weight loss in the elderly', The Journal of Nutrition, Health and Aging 12 (7); 487-491

What about calorie restriction, intermittent fasting, the fast 800 or similar popular eating plans for a longer, healthier life?

There are always new diet plans being promoted. You may have read about or heard people speak of calorie/energy restriction, 800 calorie (or kJ) plans or intermittent fasting like the 5:2 diet. All of these rely on reducing the total energy (calories or kJ) you eat, the latter on eating very little or not at all two days a week with more 'normal' eating the other five. All aim, or claim, to improve your health and possibly extend your lifespan.

Be careful: these popular plans are 'generalist'—they don't take into account the unique needs of older adults. Make no mistake, they are great for those who are younger (mid 60s or below), offering them plenty of benefits, but you must consider your own situation and age and avoid doing more harm than good.

Calorie restriction, which is not a 'diet' as such but a long-term eating philosophy, bases its claims on scientific findings that if you under-feed experimental animals (i.e. feed fewer calories/kJ than the animal would eat if food were available to them all day) for their entire adult lives, they live longer than those animals that are allowed to choose how much they eat.

Calorie restriction enthusiasts and some nutrition researchers believe the same applies to humans. There is research that shows that it may do so, and in a rural area in Japan where people eat according to the rule of 'hara hachi bu', which translates in English as 'eat only 80 percent of what you need to make you feel full', individuals commonly live healthy, active lives well into their 100s. Researchers believe the strategy of restricting calories leads to this longevity. Of course these people also live active, rural lives in smaller, supportive communities—factors very likely to be part of the picture.

Whatever the reasons, it's a virtuous plan and maybe it is the answer to long life; but one unavoidable fact remains: if you are already 65 or so IT IS TOO LATE TO START!

In order to be safe and effective, calorie restriction must be practised for as close to lifelong as possible (at least for most of an adult's life, i.e. 40 years or more). And during that time, food intake requires constant vigilance, a good understanding of nutritional science and an active lifestyle in order to get the full benefits.

For people already well into mature age—getting closer to 90 than 50—who are not already avid calorie restriction adherents, this is definitely NOT the time to take it up. Unless you are also involved in a carefully designed, fairly intensive exercise program as well (which is not easy or even advisable to take up while on a strict diet) all that is likely to happen is that you will lose out on body muscle and nutrients.

Weight reduction diets that include intermittent fasting (5:2 and similar), that encourage low energy intake for periods of time (the 'fast 800' and similar) or that have you eating all your meals in a shorter timeframe than usual (only eating between 10am and 7pm for example) have increasing following, and with good reason in younger people: it does seem that regularly challenging your body's physiology by having very limited amounts of food, none at all on some days or having a longer time without food in a 24hr timeframe can offer a number of health benefits in later life. That can mimic the way our forebears would have lived, so maybe there is something in it. In fact many of you now in your 80s and 90s probably experienced this when you were young just because of the times you lived through and it may be a contributor to your longevity.

However, timing is everything: supplying the protein,

antioxidants and other nutrients you need now and maintaining essential body muscle is difficult, if not impossible, when you have to restrict what you eat some of the time. For those of you who have very good nutritional knowledge and can plan a highly nutritious protein and nutrient-dense diet on your non-fasting days, as well as keeping up a rigorous exercise schedule to avert muscle loss, then intermittent fasting may be a good idea. But for most of you reading this, it's the same as calorie restriction: it's just too late to start.

I am lean and active—surely that's best, isn't it?

Yes, it is best! The lifestyle choices you no doubt made many years ago that made you lean and active have prepared you for a long and productive life ahead. Keep your activities up and combine them with eating the right protein and nutrients to help your body and brain counter the effects of age, and you are set.

Constant vigilance is still essential: there is no need to try to gain weight, but you must not lose it. Even though you have a better muscle reserve than most, unintentional weight loss from now on will include muscle and your health can rapidly be affected no matter how fit and well you are now.

I have always been lean but don't need to exercise to stay that way—what about me?

If you have been blessed with the ability to stay lean throughout life without needing to think too much about it and don't regularly do muscle-strengthening exercise then it might come as a surprise to learn that even a slight weight loss puts you at risk.

You may not have the risks to health that obesity imposes, and your lower weight has probably been a bonus in many ways—including making you the envy of most of your friends for years—but your muscle reserves will be less than those of a more active lean person and may be even less than those of a heavier person, so it won't take much to deplete your reserves if you should fall ill.

If you have not had to exercise much to stay lean then you're probably only a small eater, which is not always a good thing from now on. If you have even a short time being off your food or if you further cut down the amount you eat, it's going to be much harder to get what you need to support your muscles.

It's just as well, then, that it's never too late to start doing the exercise your body needs. If you do find yourself struggling to eat well at any time, be sure to act quickly to boost the nutrition in every mouthful. The tips and ideas in Foodworks will help.

I'm not overweight but not under either—am I safe?

You are safe as long as you stay active and don't allow your weight to fall. If you lose any weight, you must consciously eat and work physically to rebuild as much muscle as you can, as soon as you can. It's too easy to accept becoming less and less active with age. You have earned a rest, it's true, but at 70 and with at least a decade ahead, eating well and staying active will help those years contain the life you want them to.

I feel like I'm getting fatter—there seems to be a belly I'm sure wasn't there before.

It's sad but true that things are sliding southwards, some more than others. One reason is that the bit of fat padding, which kindly fills out the wrinkles and keeps you rounded, gradually dwindles or even changes location. You can see it go most from your face and neck, your arms and legs—and all those disappearing bottoms are further evidence of the great southern journey. Annoyingly, it tends to hang on around your middle, and no matter what you do some of the muscle lost naturally with age will be replaced by fat.

It's just not possible to do much about it diet-wise. You can keep muscle strong, and body fat at a healthy level but many healthy older people will still eventually adopt a more rounded body look with 'skinny' legs and arms. It doesn't necessarily mean you are piling on excessive fat kilos.

Even the most active person may well have a bit of a belly. Your abdominal muscles are not as strong as they were, so even with not much extra body fat you are probably going to see that belly develop. If you prided yourself when younger on being lean you might struggle more than others to accept such changes, but it's vital that you do because dieting to lose your belly might put you at risk.

Even if you are carrying a lot of excess weight around your abdomen, which is widely thought not to be good for your health no matter what your age, the same applies: dieting now to get rid of that is counterproductive. Exercise is still the key. While it may not completely get rid of that belly, strengthening abdominal muscles and staying active to boost all your body muscle is the only answer.

I have lost weight I didn't intend to lose—what should I do now?

It might not be possible now to regain all the weight or muscle you've lost, but your independence relies on you giving it your best try. It's important to act now before the situation gets worse.

That means eating enough to be able to rebuild muscle as well as putting anything you can back into storage. The rebuilding also needs you to do whatever activity you can, and it's likely both the eating and the activity will be challenging. To regain weight, particularly muscle, you need to eat more calories and more protein. That doesn't mean you have to eat huge amounts of food, but you do need to make even the smallest mouthful worth the effort. This is not normal healthy eating, it's a unique situation where most of the healthy eating advice you know gets turned on its head.

Sure, being active and getting all the exercise you need is ideal, but if you have lost weight through illness or an accident, then exercise might be a bit beyond you for a while. Make a start by eating properly first, and add activity as soon as you can.

To regain weight, what is needed now is more of a short-term 'emergency' nutrition plan than anything resembling the advice elsewhere in this book. You need extra cheese sprinkled on pasta, extra butter melted over your vegetables, extra cream on your dessert, extra chips with your meal, extra milk powder added to your drinks. You need to choose the deep-fried fish, not the grilled, and to enjoy that tail on the lamb chop, not cut it off. Say yes to the cake, the ice cream, the milkshake, the party pie and the crispy skin on the BBQ chicken. All these foods have plenty of kilojoules and many are also good suppliers of protein. And if you can't handle all that, try some of the high protein, high-energy drinks and eating suggestions in Foodworks to help you.

If you need to boost your appetite you may need to launch a dual offensive: that is, tricks (covered in Healthworks) along with strategies to make the most of what you can manage to eat (the Eating Plans in Foodworks will give you ideas).

Gerald's story

Gerald had been fairly active for most of his life and watched his weight, but he gained ten or so kilos (22lb) in his 60s. After seeing a TV commercial for some diet shakes when he was 75, he decided to give them a go to lose those extra kilos.

He was very committed to the diet shakes, and on some days even chose to have fewer than suggested. He lost ten kilos in a bit over a month, but even though he was now close to the weight he had been years before, he didn't feel as well as he had hoped.

His appetite was down, and while he thought this useful to stop him putting weight back on, he was finding he had very little interest in food at all and could only eat very small meals. He continued to lose weight even though he no longer wanted to. When his weight was down by 12 kilos (26lb), Gerald found that he wasn't able to do the things he wanted to. He had to bow out of a couple of bushwalks he was planning with friends because he felt so tired and weak and was afraid he would fall or pass out on the walk. He began to find even getting out of bed in the morning was a challenge. Then he suffered a bladder infection, which left him very unwell and weak and led to him having a fall at home. He didn't break any bones, fortunately, but was stuck in an awkward position and couldn't get himself up until a neighbour happened to come by. He had a large cut on his leg and had to have community nurses come to dress it for many weeks while it slowly healed.

Gerald didn't think his weight loss was to blame, but he was mistaken: it hadn't been good for him after all, and had hampered his independence.

What happened here?

Gerald was wrong to think that weight loss was a good idea at his age, especially such dramatic loss. It resulted in a decreased appetite, a rapid move into frailty and a reduction in his ability to heal and fight infection. Even though the diet shakes were probably high in protein, they were no doubt extremely low in calories and just not enough for him. Not only that but, without carefully planned exercise to accompany his diet, Gerald would have lost a considerable amount of muscle and that quickly affected his health, his mobility and his independence.

BODYWORKS

PART 3

Helping Your Bones to Help You.

*M*uscle is not much use to you without the skeleton it's attached to. And it might surprise you to know that bone is not a static structure, it is constantly being remodelled: much the same as muscle, maintaining them is an essential lifelong pursuit.

Bone has a soft protein framework made hard when minerals—calcium (mostly) and phosphate—are added to it, making a dense, strong structure. These minerals are also used by other body systems and can move out of bone to supply those if necessary—reducing the strength and 'bone density' so that fractures become more likely.

Calcium is needed by your heart to keep it functioning properly (among other things), with your bones acting as a store. If you don't eat enough calcium for the needs of both your bones and your heart, the extra your heart needs will be robbed from your bones.

Bone builds and strengthens when it gets the nutrients it needs, when signals from hormones tell it to do so and when the muscles attached to it work. This constant rebuilding and remodelling continues as long as removal doesn't outpace replacement.

The impacts of moving away from peak adulthood into later age for bones are similar to muscle because the physiological drivers to build your skeletal framework are no longer in play: minerals lost aren't always replaced, bone density can fall and osteoporosis develop.

Figure 8: Osteoporosis

Osteoporosis is the extreme of low bone density. It is the cause of one person being hospitalised with a fracture every hour of every day! In Australia one in every two women and one in every three men over 60 are likely to suffer a fracture due to osteoporosis. Osteoporotic bone, when viewed on an x- ray, appears to be filled with holes; it is extremely fragile. Your chances of developing it are higher if you:

> Have a family history of osteoporosis

> Don't get enough exercise

> Smoke or drink excessive amounts of alcohol

> Don't get enough calcium and vitamin D

> Take certain (steroid) medications for long periods of time.

There are many organisations providing excellent advice on avoiding and dealing with osteoporosis, some are listed at the end of this book.

Luckily your muscles help out: as they work, they 'stress' the bones by causing them to flex just a bit and that signals rebuilding. However, that can only happen when the nutrients needed to do that—predominantly protein, calcium and vitamin D—are supplied. Vitamin D does not form part of bone structure, but it is essential for the building work.

Trips and stones may break your bones!

Consider Frank.

Frank was never a big person and prided himself on his slim build. He was fiercely independent and after his wife died he was determined to cope alone in his own home 'until the end'. He was not a big exerciser at any time in his life: he played bowls after he retired and busied himself at home and in the garden, but had a gardener to do the heavier work. Since his mid 60s he had gradually lost weight, and by the time he reached his late 70s was thin but happy with that. He took no medications and continued to do most of the things he wanted to, just more slowly, and was insulted by his doctor's suggestion that he should consider a stick or other walking aid as well as further assistance at home.

Then disaster struck. One day while walking to the mailbox, Frank stumbled on the path and fell against the low brick fence. He suffered a fractured hip and a number of nasty grazes and bruises. In hospital he was found to have osteoporosis and to be vitamin D deficient. Frank was surprised: osteoporosis was something his wife had worried about, but he didn't think it would affect him. He never thought that his careful avoidance of the sun could do him any harm.

Unfortunately Frank's story isn't as hopeful as he'd like. His reduced muscle reserve along with the osteoporosis slowed his recovery after surgery, and when he did return home he needed a lot of assistance to stay there, so it wasn't long before he needed to move to a residential care home, something he had always wanted to avoid.

Could Frank have avoided his sudden loss of independence?

Certainly accidents happen, but a lot could have been done to minimise the impact of his fall so he could still be happily independent. Osteoporosis can affect men as well as women if they don't remain active and eat to support their bones.

It's no surprise to anyone that breaking a bone is bad news, but at a later age it's not only bad news, it's a potential disaster. First, there's the immobilisation while you recover, which further robs you of both bone and muscle, then the added physical assault of surgery should it be necessary (not to mention the higher risk of complications, wound infection and even death in surgery for older people), and of course the knock to your confidence and ability to move around as you did before.

Having strong bones won't stop you falling, but they might help you avoid a fracture if you do.

If you have already been diagnosed with osteoporosis there are things you can do to keep as much strength in your bones as possible, and maybe even add some. There are medical treatments and the same food rules apply whether you have osteoporosis or not. Exercise is important but check with your doctor and/or your physiotherapist before you embark because you may need a carefully designed plan to avoid causing additional damage.

Food for your bones

Calcium is what gives bone its strength. Protein forms the framework and helps absorb the calcium from foods, and vitamin D is essential for that calcium to be incorporated into the bone. You need all three to keep your bones up to scratch.

All of this is covered in greater detail in Foodworks, but two quick things. Firstly, as with most nutrients, calcium is much better tolerated by the body when you get it from food, but if you need to take a supplement, one also containing vitamin D is usually best because high dose supplements of calcium alone have been linked to heart issues. Secondly, if you avoid sun exposure due to skin cancer concerns, you must pay close attention to getting vitamin D from the limited numbers of foods containing this vitamin (check in Foodworks) and discuss with your doctor or dietitian whether you might need a supplement.

I read somewhere that eating a lot of protein causes calcium to be removed from your bones. Is that true?

This was a concern a few years ago, but it related to research into younger people eating very large amounts of protein foods with limited calcium. It's really not a problem in older people. Protein foods boost the absorption of calcium, so that makes them useful as you get older. Getting both protein and calcium is important. Dairy foods supply calcium along with protein and even some vitamin D, and they don't need to be low fat now you are older with full cream dairy foods possibly easier for the body to use.

Exercise for your bones

Exercise and activity are not just for your muscles. They are just as important to your bones, because as muscles work to move your limbs and body around they cause the bones nearby to flex just a little. This sends signals that help boost bone density and strength. Your bones, as much as your muscles, pay a high price for your declining activity levels and the limited hard

57

muscle workouts in our modern lives.

Everyday activities—moving around your home or the shops—won't help your bones sufficiently once you get into your later years. They need exercises that 'stress' them more than that. Fortunately, the same exercises that are good for your muscles also help your bones.

(The same lists of activities for your muscles given earlier in this section are also helping your bones)

To 'stress' those bones a bit in everyday life:

> Walk up stairs instead of using the lift

> Walk faster rather than slowly

> Use ankle or hand weights when you exercise.

Resistance exercise (lifting or pushing a weight with your arms, legs or whole body) and weight-bearing exercise (the type in which you actually carry your body weight) are the keys. If muscle weakens so will bone: if you are immobilised, bone is also lost. If you don't eat enough to maintain your weight, your bones will lose out too.

Medications to help your bones

There are a number of medications that can help boost your bone density and reduce osteoporosis. In later age, many medications do a lot more to help your bones than diet alone can do—but it's important to be aware that these medications must be taken strictly as directed and they require your calcium and vitamin D levels to be good at the same time.

Anyone with a slowed swallow (common in someone who is frail) or a narrowed oesophagus (the tube between your mouth and stomach) needs special consideration. This relates mostly to the bisphosphonates (Alendronate, Raloxifene, Risedronate and others with brand names in Australia including *Fosamax*™, *Actonel*™, *Skelid*™, *Didronel*™), which have been around for a while. They require you to take a tablet soon after waking, and then to sit upright for around half an hour before you eat or drink anything. If you lie down during that time, if you eat too soon or if you take the medication before bedtime, your oesophagus can become irritated and eventually it will be uncomfortable or difficult for you to swallow food.

Other medications to preserve bone density (including Densomab—brand names in Australia include *Prolia*™, *Xgeva*™, Hormone Replacement Therapy [HRT] medications or Teriparatide—brand name *Forteo*™) don't have such requirements. Check with your doctor and carefully follow the directions on any prescribed medications.

BODYWORKS

PART 4

Born to Move: Exercise and Activity for Life

The importance of exercise

I know you are going to get tired of me saying it, but here I go again: there is no choice but to stay active and get all the exercise you can. Physical activity does a number of great things for your body and your brain. It assists with glucose metabolism and diabetes management and reduces insulin resistance; it reduces chronic inflammation, maximises blood flow through the body and brain, helps build and support both new and old brain cell connections (increasing brain plasticity) and more.

Minimise immobility at all costs

Of course relaxation is vital for good health, but our sedentary lives increase the inflammation you will read so much about in this book. It's too easy to find excuses to slump instead of sit up straight, sit when we could stand, drive when we could walk, take the lift when we could make the effort to walk up the stairs. Earlier in this section I touched on how research carried out with astronauts in zero gravity has shown that removing the influence of gravity on the body results in muscle and bone loss and increases inflammation.

None of us are experiencing zero gravity, but in later life, when the hormones and nerves that signal the building of muscle and bone are out of the picture, the effect of being immobile is very similar to what astronauts face. The old fashioned 'bed rest' recommended in illness and injury needs to be kept to a minimum for your body and your brain. Sure, rest when it's needed, but as soon as you can, sit up, stand up, get out of bed. Work against gravity at every opportunity. Every minute you are active or doing something helps reduce inflammation. No matter what you weigh, if you spend less time watching TV, sitting at the computer or in an armchair, driving in the car or sitting on a bus and more time being up and about, you will help your body and your brain.

There are great resources at the end of this section, which you can access to help stay as active as possible.

Here I want to give you some guidance on the basics.

First off, if you haven't done much exercise for a while, check with your doctor and be aware that exercising while you are ill might do you harm so take care. It's usually okay if you are recovering from an accident or surgery—the sooner you can move those muscles and bones the better—but not if you are actually suffering an illness.

The basics:

> Warm up/cool down on either side of activity

> Gradually build up resistance and intensity

> Do things that make you puff and/or sweat a bit.

Next, plan your exercises!

To avoid overuse causing you excess pain, use different muscle groups on different days. It's best to use one or two major muscle groups each time you do strength exercises. Then after a couple of days work a different group. Allow at least a few days between repeating an activity in the same muscle group.

Aerobic activities like walking, jogging, cycling, swimming and sport activities use a wide range of muscles and won't usually require these considerations, although you do have to work up the length of time you spend on each.

You need to do physical exercise regularly: combine aerobic activities like walking (or anything that makes you puff) with things that make your muscles work hard enough so you feel them. Walking is usually not enough. If you play a sport, do activities such as rowing, extensive bushwalking or cycling that combine strength activity with aerobics; that is the ideal. Gym work is a good option if it combines strength work with balance and aerobic activity.

Gentle exercises are all some people will be able to manage and anything is better than inactivity, but these are best seen as a starting point. Build on the gentle exercises (ideally under the guidance of a qualified exercise professional) as soon as you can to gain strength and ability.

You should expect to feel mild muscle soreness in the days after exercise, but as you get used to each activity that will fade. If there is any severe pain, stop that exercise and check with your doctor, physiotherapist or professionally qualified exercise professional.

Get out of the chair, stop leaning on handrails, get up off the floor

I think it's worthwhile doing everyday muscle work that gives you extra benefits. Getting out of your chair just using muscle work, negotiating stairs or ramps while staying as upright as possible and getting up from the floor are three things to work on. It's far too easy to get in the habit of always pushing yourself out of your chair using its arms and leaning heavily on a bannister or handrail on stairs or ramps and of course getting down to the floor might be far too simple. How you do the first two might allow the last to be accomplished with some sort of grace instead of a thud.

All of these boost muscle strength by just challenging gravity, but getting your body from the ground to upright uses so many muscle groups its extra beneficial. And, if you do end up on the floor (hopefully having avoided a fracture) being able to get up again is an immensely valuable skill to have!

Some will need to take the chair and the handrail very slowly—perhaps starting with working on getting out of your chair without using the arms of the chair to push off. When you take the stairs or negotiate a ramp the handrail is important so you can stop yourself falling, but gradually try to reduce the pressure you need to apply to do that. Stand as straight as you can, pushing your sternum (the flat bone covering your heart attached to your ribs) up and forward and gradually lighten the pressure you apply to the handrail. After a time you may be able to hover your hand over the rail so it's in place to grab hold should you miss your footing, but you are not relying on it to pull you up the stairs or to lean on going down.

When it comes to getting up off the floor, I need to stress the importance of trying it first with someone close by to make sure you make it up safely! When you do have support to give it a go, if it's been a long time since you have intentionally been on the floor, it's certainly not an easy progress fighting gravity to get back up at first. Take it slowly, in stages, using sturdy furniture to assist until you build up strength. The more you practice that, the stronger the muscles used to get you upright will become.

Resistance exercise: bands and weights

Resistance bands are flexible elasticised bands that are wrapped round your hands while you do activities to help you work against the resistance they present. Your exercise professional can instruct you how to use them. You can purchase 500g or 1kg hand or ankle weights (or heavier) but you can also use everyday items such as cans of soup or even bags of shopping. With both, it's essential to start slowly with the lowest weight you need. That may be no weight at all, then work up to heavier weights as you progress. To be assured you are gaining benefit, each activity should feel challenging and even a bit hard.

The weight is too heavy if you can't repeat the exercise eight times. You should then drop back until your muscles have become accustomed to a lower weight. Aim to be able to repeat each exercise 10 to 15 times. When you can do those easily you can add more weight if you wish.

Don't move too fast and don't drop your weights quickly. A rule of thumb is to count to three as you lift, push or pull; hold for one count, then take two counts to return to rest. Always breathe out as you lift, push or pull, and breathe in as you return to rest.

Bodyworks

Take home from this section:

> Exercise, exercise, exercise—whatever you can do

> Protein at every meal—extra if you have been unwell or need to rebuild

> Whatever you weigh now, stay active but don't aim to lose weight without a very good exercise plan.

BRAINWORKS

PART 1

The Active Brain

Everything that applies to your muscles also holds true for your brain: keep it active and feed it properly.

An active brain means you'll continue to engage in spirited conversation, prepare and savour great meals, enjoy music and books, decide if a piece of art is worth the canvas it's painted on, plan and accomplish every day tasks, judge the safety and appropriateness of everything you do whether it's walking along a beach, doing the shopping, driving a car or playing tennis, and allow you to keep on track with the people and the world around you.

Keeping all that up and reducing your risk of dementia is about more than doing Sudoku or learning Russian: all the things you do to stay physically active are just as important, probably more so. It's easy to see how physical activity keeps your brain working while coordinating tennis shots or negotiating the varied terrain of a bushwalk, but the physical activity you do also keeps blood flowing through your brain as well as providing many other benefits we've already touched on and will come back to over and over.

Very hungry, very demanding

Your brain is only about 2% of your body weight but that tiny control centre uses 20 to 25% of the energy and commandeers between 15 and 20% of the blood flow in the entire body at any time. It has so much more going on given the space it occupies than anywhere else in the body: impressive for sure, but that fantastic level of activity also makes it extra demanding on fuel and resources and vulnerable to even tiny amounts of damage.

If that fuel or those other resources the brain needs are not there where and when needed, or if even the tiniest amount of damage occurs, that can create an inflammatory response in the brain. Inflammation is necessary in the body, but it needs to be well controlled to be safe. When I mention it in the context of the brain, I am referring to inflammation that exceeds that control. That sort of inflammation must be minimised for your brain's sake.

Neurons and plasticity

The brain has a lot to do and communication is central. More than 80 billion neurons (also called neurones or nerve cells) form an intricate network, with each neuron able to connect with many more, all passing messages using neurotransmitter chemicals between themselves and other nerves coming in from the body and going away from the brain. The network develops and is refined with learning and experience throughout life. The more connections made, the greater flexibility your brain has to keep you engaged with the world around you.

No matter your age, training and practice keep neurons active and encourage the building of extra connections as needed. Even when some connections have been severed, blocked or damaged by injury or trauma, they can often be 'rewired' to bypass the blockage: this ability to re-route networks is called plasticity and gives the brain some flexibility to adapt even after significant damage has occurred.

To make new connections and to maintain plasticity, the brain relies on a number of chemicals, including brain derived neurotrophic factor or BDNF (the name means 'a substance the brain makes that is able to grow new neurons', so it makes sense). The way we live, including how active we are in life and to some extent what we eat, influences the availability of BDNF. Depression, anxiety and stress all tend to reduce BDNF availability, while physical activity balanced by meditative practice and relaxation tend to increase it: you know what you need to do!

Setting you up for good brain capacity: the power of cognitive reserve

Life provides the brain with more than a way to show off its skills: every new learning experience, every challenge mastered, every skill practiced and honed, all the ways we dare our brains to do new things forces it to set up more and more complex internal networks—making more and more connections between individual cells.

This gives us what's called cognitive reserve and it's rather like road access into a small town: if there is only a single road in and out of town and the bridge over the river on that road is destroyed by flood, traffic flow is going to stop completely. If there is an alternate route up a steep, windy back road then it's possible to get to town but traffic will slow down a bit. If there is a network of roads in the area, then it's just a matter of using an alternate route and might not cause much delay at all.

That's how cognitive reserve is built and works: the more experience the brain gets, the bigger the network of connections it develops and the more chance that it will be able to use alternate routes to continue carrying out complex tasks for many years, even if occasional 'roadblocks' occur.

Having a higher cognitive reserve—and that can be increased at any time in life—helps reduce the risk of developing dementia and helps people manage their lives better for longer if they do encounter cognitive issues.

Setting you up for good brain health: the bonus of an active life lived

If you are now in your late 70s or beyond, you are at a decided advantage cognition-wise, because you grew up when life was less sedentary than it is for most now: walking long distances to school, being shooed outside most of the day, and with plenty of labour intensive chores to do each day. We are designed to be physically active our entire lives and unfortunately doing less than we should day in and day out has many effects on the brain, especially inflammation, as you will read.

MAINTENANCE AND LOGISTICS: SUPPLYING WHAT'S NEEDED, ELIMINATING WHAT'S NOT.

Blood supply

All these clever and complex systems cannot achieve anything unless they are fed, watered and protected. The blood handles the logistics of delivering everything the brain needs. It carries nutrients from the gut and oxygen from the lungs to cells throughout the body and brain and removes waste in the same way.

It's highly efficient at accomplishing all those tasks and it needs to be: neurons are more sensitive to oxygen deprivation than other cells. Body cells can often survive short disruption to blood flow and oxygen supply, but neurons can't, they can be irreparably damaged or die if blood flow is restricted and not corrected quickly.

Blood vessels inside the brain also work a little differently compared to the body. While substances in body blood vessels can generally move directly between blood and cells, delivery into brain cells (and out) for some things, including glucose and the amino acid building blocks of BDNF and neurotransmitters, require negotiating a specialised system: the blood-brain-barrier.

This barrier acts as a security cordon for the highly vulnerable neurons to stop toxins gaining access, but like many security cordons, it can slow the movement of what you want to get in or out.

There are a few substances small enough to slip through the blood-brain-barrier unnoticed, but many important ones need to access special 'carrier' systems, which act like VIP passes to usher them across.

Agility

agility: the ability to move quickly and easily, nimbleness

The logistics operation needs to be agile as well as efficient.

Delivering resources immediately to the specific area of the brain doing whatever task is happening at any point in time requires blood flow to instantly be ramped up through that area. This is how humans can accomplish both very basic and immensely challenging tasks every day.

At any moment, large parts of your brain are doing day-to-day tasks like maintaining your breathing and heartbeat and keeping your organs functioning. Tasks that if you had to actually think about, would leave you no time in the day, but without them you wouldn't be alive. These tasks use about the same amount of resources and produce the same amount of waste each day, so the amount of blood that needs to pass through the areas involved doesn't need to fluctuate dramatically to keep them in working order.

This is not the case in areas managing complex information, when detailed planning and thinking need to be done or when you need to assess how to respond in a situation, relate to another person, find your way in a new environment, learn or remember something or an endless array of other complex processing tasks.

While the parts of the brain that carry out these tasks are never silent, they can be quiet—during rest times—but need to rev up to allow you just to speak or read and must increase dramatically for more complex activities. They need more resources right away so you can keep up and they need rapid, efficient removal of waste products to avoid long-term damage.

The quiet achievers: glia and other neuron supporters

That's where cells called glia come in: these fabulous cells (comprising a number of different groups including astrocytes) outnumber neurons—some say by eight times or more—and have vital roles we already know of and more than likely others we are yet to discover.

It is the glia that trigger ramping up blood flow into the areas doing the extra work, so it's not surprising that there are more of them where complex thought and planning happen compared to parts that do more routine tasks. They also help protect the brain by seeking out and removing dead and damaged cells and assist in communication between neurons.

If they are not working as they should, especially if their capacity to increase blood flow is hampered at all, not only are you likely to struggle with complex processing and thought but blood flow restriction can trigger inflammation with longer term impacts and associated cell damage.

A vast network of blood vessels and a brain-specific lymph system called the glymphatic system support glia.

Deep cleaning: the glymphatic system

Every time something happens in the brain, some sort of waste is produced and it must be removed to avoid causing damage.

We have known for decades that blood and the cerebrospinal fluid that bathes the brain carry out this removal process, but researchers have always been puzzled by exactly how they manage it for a few reasons. First, the brain is so metabolically active (a medical term meaning it does a lot of stuff) that more waste is produced than these have capacity to manage. Secondly, cerebrospinal fluid flow out of the brain was known to be limited—little more than a trickle—and the blood-brain-barrier restricts the quantities of waste product that are able to be cleared, especially at times of high activity.

It was only in 2012 that an advance in brain imaging resulted in the discovery of the beautiful brain-specific lymph system, now called the glymphatic system. The glia manage this system, which uses an awe-inspiring network of microscopic channels running throughout the brain moving cerebrospinal fluid under pressure, collecting brain activity waste products and whisking them away from the cells before they can cause any damage. As with most things, the glymphatic system doesn't work alone, it depends on blood flow through the brain. If blood is not flowing, the glymphatic system can't work. If blood flow is restricted in any way, its work is hampered: the harmful effects of temporary or partial restriction to blood flow over many years, including inflammation, cannot be understated. You will read more on this and its potential impacts later in this chapter.

A fun fact about the glymphatic system is it seems it is especially active while you sleep, so you might think those hours under the blankets are just indulgence, but valuable work is being done while you are there.

BRAINWORKS

PART 2

Brain Resourcing: Fuel, Fluids, Nutrients.

GIVING YOUR BRAIN WHAT IT NEEDS
FOR ITS BEST WORK

Just as they do in the rest of your body, the food you eat and the air you breathe provide all the biochemical building blocks your brain requires to fuel its every action and to create the substances it needs to maintain itself. These building blocks are fuel, fluids and the nutrients required to build and maintain cells and brain activity.

Fuel supply

Glucose is your brain's preferred fuel. You already know how demanding the brain is for energy and to fulfil that demand it needs a constant supply of glucose to do the basics to keep you ticking along—engage in complex tasks and that demand escalates rapidly.

Increases in blood flow can get extra glucose to areas of the brain doing the work when demand goes up. However, brain cells then need to be able to get hold of the glucose using the specialised carriers to get it across the blood-brain-barrier, and the neurons and glia need to use it effectively and there are influences from insulin resistance in this as you will read later in this section.

If anything affects the efficient supply of glucose—if there is inadequate supply from food or reserves, if blood flow doesn't increase adequately to get it where it's needed, if any of the glucose carriers don't do their job, if insulin resistance is in play—the brain's ability can be impacted, especially when demand is high.

Omega-3 fats also play a part in fuelling the brain. They can't be used as fuel themselves like glucose is, but the omega-3 fat known as DHA helps neurons access and use glucose and assists the brain in many other ways. Research has shown the brains of people with Alzheimer's have lower levels of DHA and use less glucose than those without Alzheimer's, so there is a link although the full picture is yet to be understood.

The other two omega-3 fats also seem to be important: ALA and EPA are both involved in bolstering fuel supplies to cells, either by supporting glucose availability or by boosting the supply of ketones inside the brain (more on them soon) to help if glucose isn't in adequate supply.

You can read more on omega-3 fats and where to get them in Foodworks.

When fuel supply isn't sufficient

I have mentioned that the areas of the brain affected in people with Alzheimer's routinely use less glucose (and therefore achieve less) than those of other people, and it has been widely assumed that this was a result of damage caused by the disease. But it could well be the reverse: many now believe that a reduced ability to fuel brain cells actually leads to brain changes that can eventually manifest in Alzheimer's and possibly other dementias.

Not only are under-fuelled cells unable to do what you need them to, they also become more susceptible to oxidative stress, inflammation and the build-up of substances like βamyloid. If that then causes damage, a vicious cycle can start, driving worsening glucose use and more damage.

How diabetes comes into the picture: is there type 3 diabetes?

With the recognition that there is a link between glucose use in the brain and dementia there has been understandable interest in the part diabetes might play and some have suggested the term 'type 3 diabetes' is appropriate, although not everyone agrees. This idea has come about because people with type 1, type 2 and pre-diabetes (or insulin resistance) have a higher likelihood of encountering dementia later in life. There are some extremely complex factors involved in this.

Be aware that even though there is a statistically higher risk of dementia if you have diabetes, that does not mean everyone with diabetes will develop it. Like anyone else, there is a lot you can do to reduce that risk: what you eat, how you live and the activity you do remain just as important to you as someone without diabetes.

Diabetes and the different way it needs to be considered in later age is discussed in detail in Healthworks. Here we will take a brief look at how the different types of diabetes play out when it comes to the brain and dementia.

Type 1 diabetes:

People with this mostly lifelong form of diabetes need a constant supply of insulin delivered by injection or the newer pump/implant devices. In this type of diabetes, both high blood glucose levels (hyperglycaemia) and the opposite when levels fall below what the brain can tolerate (hypoglycaemia) are problematic.

Hypoglycaemia is generally more obvious, causing symptoms including confusion, disorientation and potential loss of consciousness, all of which can cause long-term issues in the brain. In fact, researchers believe that experiencing more than three or four serious hypoglycaemic events (those that are bad enough to require assistance from others) a year may cause damage to brain cells, which over many years, accumulates to increase the risk of dementia developing later in life.

We will come back to hyperglycaemia soon.

Type 2 diabetes and insulin resistance (also called pre-diabetes):

While type 2 diabetes and insulin resistance are not the same, they have similar links with dementia so I will look at them together.

Both can occur at any time in life but are more likely in adulthood and especially in people who are sedentary and/or overweight. Hypoglycaemia is less of an issue for most people because only some types of medications people with type 2 diabetes take can cause it. Rarely, if at all, will most people with type 2 or insulin resistance encounter problematic low blood glucose levels.

What is a bigger problem for the brain is blood glucose levels being chronically higher than ideal. High blood glucose levels (hyperglycaemia) are an issue for the brain in all types of diabetes because they can impact blood vessels, potentially restricting the flow of blood to and through the brain.

Insulin resistance (which is also a part of type 2) creates its own problems for the brain because, as well as its association with glucose, insulin is involved in memory, communication between brain cells and in keeping neurones healthy (including having a role in transporting βamyloid out of the brain) so insulin resistance can impact memory, neuronal communication and contribute to βamyloid build up.

Finally, recent research suggests that low-grade inflammation due to type 2 diabetes causes accumulation of a protein called tau, which indicates probable neuronal damage and is also implicated in dementia.

What is so dangerous about hypoglycaemia?

Hypoglycaemia—commonly called a 'hypo'—refers to your blood glucose level falling low enough that your brain cannot function properly. This generally happens at levels below 4 mmol/l or 72mg/dl in most people, but it can occur at higher levels in later age. As blood glucose levels fall towards the lowest your brain can tolerate, you usually get a number of warning symptoms that something is amiss, such as tingling in your face or arms and legs, vision changes, confusion, reduced coordination and a cold sweat. These warnings act as alerts, and as long as you quickly get some glucose in from food, your levels will rise and you will soon return to normal. If you don't heed these warnings, eventually your brain will 'shut you down' and you'll lose consciousness.

Unfortunately in later age and especially when you have had diabetes for many years, your ability to sense lowering glucose levels can diminish so you don't know to supply extra glucose and you can lose consciousness without the usual warning symptoms.

Why hyperglycaemia (even slightly elevated blood glucose) is such a problem

It might seem like having a bit of extra glucose in the blood will help your brain, but sadly it's the opposite.

Any blood glucose levels above normal (also often associated with insulin resistance) increase inflammation, contribute to the production of oxidative wastes, upset the fine balance in a number of systems in the brain, impact the health of blood vessels and importantly contribute to the accumulation of toxic advanced glycation end products (AGEs). All can drive accumulation of βamyloid and altered tau protein and other brain changes in dementia.

AGEs warrant more discussion because they can be quite harmful. They are substances that occur in foods and that can be made in the body from otherwise harmless glucose or other sugar molecules and protein fragments.

All of us produce these and many foods contain them and you will see from the list in figure 9 below, that they are what make many foods really yummy. The solution to minimising their potential impact is not a knee-jerk one of just stopping enjoying those foods altogether; it's about avoiding getting too many from food. It's interesting that many high AGE foods are also the highly processed foods that should be kept to a minimum.

Foods and Advanced Glycation End Products (AGEs)

The relationship between AGE levels in foods and their possible health impacts is not as straightforward as measuring what individual foods contain: there are complex interactions between individual foods, foods combined together in a meal and how they may be absorbed from foods. Being aware of foods that have higher measured levels can give you a guide.

Any cooking or processing of any food that causes browning and crisping of foods will develop AGEs, including BBQing, roasting, grilling (broiling), baking and deep frying. Foods high in protein are especially vulnerable when they also contain sugars or carbohydrates, or those are added during processing.

AGE production is reduced by addition of acids (lemon juice, vinegar) in cooking and when not dry cooked (casseroles, soups).

Figure 9: Some foods AGE contents compared:

> Chicken skin, fried meats or poultry, grilled burgers are high AGE

> BBQ, grilled or roast meat, poultry are high AGE; casseroled or stewed lower.

> Processed meats, especially when grilled or fried (crispy bacon) are high: moist cooked lower

> Commercial pizza and fast food burgers are high AGE

> Raw or steamed fish is low in AGE, levels increase with hotter, drier cooking.

> Most soy and similar foods are low AGE but that increases due to browning during cooking

> Most natural cheese is lower, processed cheese and well-aged hard cheeses are higher

> Roasted nuts and snack foods are higher in AGEs

> Potatoes are low AGE; fries and crisps are high

> Most breads, fruits and vegetables are low AGE.

Our body production is increased when blood glucose levels are higher than normal. Their impact is fortunately balanced by antioxidants, but if enough AGEs are produced or eaten and the food you choose is low in antioxidants, that capacity can be overwhelmed.

If AGEs accumulate, they can increase levels of βamyloid and affect the capacity of the brain to coordinate many things, particularly appetite and memory. They can also impact the gut microbiome by increasing 'leakiness' in the gut wall, causing intestinal inflammation and negatively impacting microbial diversity, all of which can affect the brain.

These substances do sound scary and they certainly can be because there will always be some production and some coming in from food, but most of what you already know is good for your brain also helps you detoxify AGEs and it is that capacity that is most important.

When it comes to food, it's the more highly processed, deep fried, crispy and browned foods—often common in major fast food outlets—that are the biggest problem. I go on about eating foods that have undergone as little processing as possible for a reason. If you do an internet search for AGEs you will read about the damage done by cooking meats at high temperatures (particularly BBQ). What many people don't realise is that raw meats contain virtually none, while many raw plant foods are high in AGEs (including vegetables) and they increase in both with processing. High protein foods like meat, but also any food that is treated at high temperatures and that browns as it cooks, develop AGEs. It is better to cook foods from fresh, so you can adjust the cooking method than to buy take away or ultra processed foods over which you have much less control.

It's all about balance—the AGEs in plant foods, if they do impact once we eat them, are most likely balanced by their antioxidants and phytochemicals and those same foods help minimise any impacts of AGEs from animal foods. Interestingly, one substance that researchers have found to be particularly effective in reducing the production of AGEs in the body is carnosine, which is found exclusively in the muscle of animals, so avoiding all meat may not be the answer either.

There is a lot still to learn about AGEs, but there are two things to remember. Firstly, any damage they might cause is the result of accumulation over many years. And secondly, high blood glucose is a contributor to increased problems so keeping that in line, especially in younger or middle age is important.

Staying on the straight and narrow

Before I leave diabetes, I need to mention how much the brain appreciates smooth sailing when it comes to blood glucose. Not only do both high and low blood glucose present problems, but it thrives on blood glucose levels staying as constant and predictable as possible: not swinging between too high and too low. This is because big fluctuations in blood glucose during the day trigger inflammation and we know how bad that is! Fluctuations can come about due to over-adjusting by eating too much carbohydrate after a hypo (hypoglycaemic event), or overeating because you fear a hypo might come along.

If glucose use is down, can fuel supply be boosted? Why you might hear about ketones

The brain always needs glucose, but to access a small amount of backup fuel it can use substances called ketones. However, supplying these to the cells where they could be used has its challenges.

You don't get ketones from food and they are not as simple to make in the body as glucose. We have always known that the liver makes ketones from body fat or from the fat in food. This produces worthwhile quantities only when a person is starving (and I mean really starving, not just complaining loudly of hunger!).

During starvation (or in extended fasts or extreme 'ketogenic' diets designed to mimic starvation) the brain demands fuel as always. It quickly uses up the limited glucose supplies and muscle protein is converted into glucose to add to those, but eventually, with no more food coming in, that isn't enough. The cells in the rest of the body can use body fat in the form of fatty acids to fuel their activities but the brain can't. So, the liver swings into action, converting fatty acids into ketones, which can be used under these extreme circumstances to add to the glucose coming from muscle protein to fuel hungry brain cells.

This is good, because the brain can function with ketones as a supplementary fuel. BUT (yes, there is often a 'but') brain cells that for whatever reason are under-using glucose and might benefit from a regular supply of ketones to help out are not going to get them unless you are actually starving, because the liver doesn't normally make them.

There has been a lot of interest in manipulating the diet to get the liver to make more ketones to boost brain capacity when it's not using glucose as well as it should. Diets that push the liver to produce ketones are called ketogenic. They are not new. In the past they've been used in two main ways: in weight loss, because they encourage the use of body fat, but they are pretty extreme and often don't achieve long-term success as the resumption of a more usual diet frequently results in weight regain.

Their other use has been in treating severe epilepsy in children, and it is from this use, recognising that ketones can affect brain function, that they come into our discussion here. Logic says that if ketogenic diets can help in a brain condition like epilepsy, and the brains of those with cognitive decline and dementia might benefit from an extra supply of ketones, maybe this is an answer. Researchers started to look at using these diets to boost cognition in people with cognitive decline and dementia but the findings haven't been as good as hoped. One huge issue is that strict ketogenic diets are not easy for anyone to manage and people already living with dementia generally find them too unusual and challenging to achieve.

So the strict ketogenic diet was modified using a type of fat called medium chain triglyceride (MCT). This is a really interesting fat because it's able to bypass the conversion into fatty acids that other fats have to go through before they can be made into ketones in the liver. Because MCTs can be converted directly into ketones it was thought they might be a big plus when brain glucose use was down. This newer modified ketogenic diet doesn't require the severe restriction of carbohydrate foods, so was considered a bit easier to manage.

The most abundant source of MCTs in food is coconut or coconut oil, which is now widely marketed in organic, virgin and all manner of other forms, but was copha in my childhood chocolate crackle-making days! MCTs are now also supplied in commercial oil preparations. Manufacturers of these oils and coconut products widely promoted the benefits of the MCT diet in treating dementia a few years ago, even claiming preventive abilities.

There really is only anecdotal evidence to support their claims— meaning a small number of people said it worked for them— and unfortunately, it's not the universal cure it was hoped to be. Also, taking on a high coconut oil diet can cause diarrhoea and it is a highly saturated fat with a negative impact on heart and blood vessel health.

Recently, advanced technology in neuroscience has produced a revelation about ketones: the astrocytes (a type of glia) in the brain are able to make ketones themselves unrelated to anything you might eat. Because glia assist neurons in so many ways, their providing this supply of ketones inside the brain might be one way they help maintain brain health. When astrocytes are affected by inflammation or oxidative stress they might lose some or all of that ability.

There is a long way to go in our understanding of this whole area, but certainly doing all that is possible to help astrocytes—the same as supporting every other cell in the body—reducing oxidative stress and chronic inflammation is a better bet than taking on the latest fad.

Fluid supply

Your brain cannot fire on all cylinders when you are even a little bit dehydrated, no matter your age. And if dehydration worsens it can present almost insurmountable challenges, bringing on confusion and incoherence surprisingly quickly—and that gets more likely as you get older.

Without adequate hydration, neurons can't communicate with each other, which after all is what cognition is all about. Dehydration also slows down blood flow through the brain, not only directly impacting fuel/nutrient delivery and the glymphatic system, but also resulting in the release of stress hormones. Excessive levels of these cause inflammation, affect the production of neurotransmitters and mess up the actions not only of the neurons themselves but also of the glial cells, leaving them unable to support and protect the neurons, as they should.

If you become unwell, even mild dehydration makes delirium far more likely—and that is a significant issue for your brain (read more on delirium later in this section).

Even when you know all this, good hydration is often a challenge because as you grow older you don't feel thirsty as soon as you should. That happens for a lot of reasons (summarised in figure

10 below), but basically it is because the mechanisms that monitor hydration levels and send you messages to drink are affected by ageing—the messages don't get through. Feeling thirsty becomes a less useful measure of fluid needs as you move into your later years.

It is common among people moving into their later years to actively avoiding drinking, especially as evening approaches, aiming to reduce the need to get up during the night to have a wee. However, this often has the opposite effect. Drinking less than you need increases the concentration of the urine, which irritates the bladder, causing it to send signals to empty much more frequently. You may need to get up more often even though not much comes out at each visit to the toilet.

Some of the messages about thirst are combined with messages about hunger, so if your appetite for food declines, you may not get the messages to drink either. (Appetite, how it changes and what you can do about it are covered in detail in Healthworks).

If you do eat less food for any reason, the amount of fluid available to your body and brain also reduces, because a lot of the water our bodies get each day comes from the food we eat and from the digestive process itself as foods are broken down.

We do hold some fluid reserves in our bodies that can provide temporary backup, but they are held largely in body muscle. If you have lost weight, and therefore muscle, since your late 60s you have also reduced that reserve and need to be extra vigilant.

Figure 10:

> **Factors contributing to increased chance of dehydration in older people:**
>
> Changes in the kidney's ability to retain water due to:
>
> > ❯ Altered hormone levels
> >
> > ❯ Age-related loss of kidney function.
>
> Decreased sense of thirst
>
> Diarrhoea or frequent loose motions (often resulting in reduced food/liquid intake)
>
> Urinary incontinence and subsequent avoidance of drinking to reduce chance of accident.
>
> Cognitive impairment and dementia

Diuretic medications (fluid tablets)

Diuretics (commonly called fluid tablets) are designed to remove excess fluid from your body, to relieve some of the symptoms of heart problems. Keeping a balance between too much fluid affecting your heart and having enough to keep the rest of your body functioning is something that needs close monitoring by your doctor. It's essential to be aware that the dosage of the medications required can vary with weight loss and changes in your health, so don't assume you always need the same dose. If you are unwell—especially with a fever—or heading for surgery adjustments may need to be made until you have recovered to avoid delirium and dehydration.

Medications that can play a part in hydration/dehydration:

The brand names of diuretics include *Lasix, Frusemide*

Other medications that can contribute to dehydration:

> ❯ Laxatives—too numerous to specify brands

> ❯ ACE inhibitor blood pressure medications—Australian brand names include *Coversyl, Tritace, Ramace, Indosyl, Monopril, Capoten, Renitec, Gopten*

> ❯ Steroids

> ❯ Antipsychotics—includes *Chlorpromazine, Haloperidol, Clozapine, Risperidone, Olanzapine.*

Neurotransmitter supply—food and more

I'm not going to discuss what's needed to build brain cells—neurons and glia—because they are generally like every other body cell, but the brain does need to make some things specific to its needs, particularly neurotransmitters. There are well over 100 different substances that do this role. Some are present in food we eat but it is unclear whether those survive being broken down during the digestive process and if they do, what influence they might have on the other side of the blood-brain-barrier, inside the b rain.

Neurotransmitters – a glimpse of what a few do and where they come from

All neurotransmitters are made in both the brain and the gut. There are also some in the foods we eat although currently we don't know what influence, if any, they might have—they may be changed or be broken down during digestion for one thing. There are a few food sources mentioned here mainly for interest, but overall any benefits they offer could just as well be from their wider capacity to promote good gut health.

Serotonin is involved in mood with ideal levels in the brain tending to result in a positive outlook and low anxiety and stress. As a result, it's the target of the most common antidepressants, the SSRIs (selective serotonin reuptake inhibitors), but it also has important roles in memory, learning, sleep and social behaviour. Gut bacteria produce more than 90% of your serotonin and while gut-produced serotonin doesn't travel to the brain directly, its production in the gut certainly influences the brain in many ways. A healthy gut microbiome is associated with increased serotonin levels in the brain and better cognition.

Some foods that contain serotonin are: bananas, Chinese cabbage, hazelnut, kiwi, lettuce, nettle, paprika, passionfruit, pawpaw, pepper, pineapple, pomegranate, potato, spinach, strawberry and tomato.

GABA supports mental alertness and mood by reducing the number of nerve signals happening at any one time (having an inhibitory effect). That might sound like a bad thing but it's vital because keeping the brain on track depends on being in control and either too many or too few nerve signals cause problems. A lack of GABA leaves your central nervous system with too many signals and causes conditions like epilepsy, seizures or mood disorders involving aggressive behaviour. Meanwhile, too much GABA means not enough brain activity and can lead to hypersomnia (daytime sleepiness) and low mood.

GABA supplements are commonly promoted on the internet and by some vocal enthusiasts—these are claimed to reduce anxiety and help people sleep. These, and related medications (including many common sedatives like valium and alcohol) aim to increase the effects of GABA. Some care needs to be taken with these, especially at later age, because they can take some time to leave the body and prolong drowsiness and lack of coordination so the risk of falls increase. Prescribed medications are carefully balanced to your individual needs, while supplements are less predictable. Always tell your doctor if you decide to take a GABA supplement, no matter how 'natural' it sounds, including herbs such as St John's Wort and valerian, which have impacts on GABA.

Again, production by gut bacteria has an important role to play and some is found in foods (although you have to eat a lot for that to be significant). They include foods the gut bacteria love—most pulses and whole grains as well as spinach, potato and sweet potato.

Dopamine is involved in control of the brain's reward and pleasure centres as well as in regulating movement, emotional responses, competitiveness and aggression. This is the neurotransmitter impacted in Parkinson's disease where inadequate supply most obviously causes movement issues, but a type of dementia can also develop over time in Parkinson's. In contrast an oversupply (that happens when taking some illicit drugs, particularly methamphetamines) causes excessive emotional responses including euphoria, but also severe aggression. It is also produced by neurons in the gut wall, being involved in immunity and the inflammatory response including in inflammatory bowel disease.

Dopamine is made in the brain from the amino acid tyrosine and its production by neurons in the gut wall is influenced by the health of the gut microbiome. It is contained in some foods including aubergine (eggplant), avocado, banana, common bean, apple, orange, pea, spinach and tomato.

Digestion breaks protein into its basic components (amino acids), which can be used to make different neurotransmitters inside and out of the brain. Neurotransmitters don't only work in the brain, they are also made by the gut bacteria, facilitating communication between them, impacting the working of the digestive tract and potentially influencing the brain via the vague nerve, which links the gut and the brain.

Neurotransmitters circulating in the blood are generally unable to cross the blood-brain-barrier, so the brain needs to make its own from amino acid building blocks that can get across. Amino acids get across the blood-brain-barrier with assistance from their own transporters, but there are issues. Different combinations of the 20 amino acids make up different neurotransmitters, but the transport systems don't necessarily align exactly with what is needed inside brain cells.

I liken the situation for amino acids to a car ferry on a river crossing: there are only a certain number of ferries so the number of vehicles (amino acids) that can get across at any one time is limited and the ferry operators don't play favourites between different types of vehicle—it's a first-in line, first on system. So even though brain cells may be waiting on the other side for specific amino acids to make specific neurotransmitters, the ones they need have to wait in line with other amino acids being ferried over for different tasks. It's not hard to see how easily that can impact production of individual neurotransmitters, especially at times when needs are high.

You may have heard about foods or supplements you can eat to influence mood or behaviour. In 2019 the most commonly promoted contained the neurotransmitter GABA or gamma-Aminobutyric acid, claimed to promote relaxation and sleep.

Others include the amino acid tryptophan, which is needed to make serotonin and is claimed to help reduce depression.

The idea of supplements containing individual amino acids is that by providing those required to make particular neurotransmitters, you encourage the brain to make more of them. However, the blood-brain-barrier gets in the way of that, literally and figuratively, because unless you eat nothing but the supplement itself, the amino acids it contains will need to queue for the ferry along with all the others from protein foods you have eaten. There is no guarantee that the ones you want right away will make it across more quickly than others.

Unfortunately, studies that prove the claims made by supplement manufacturers are mixed and where they do suggest possible benefits, there is no answer yet exactly how they work, which makes long-term benefits unclear.

What research is increasingly showing is the involvement of the gut microbiome (the community of gut bacteria). Not only do gut bacteria themselves produce neurotransmitters, the microbiome is also able to influence the production of others inside the brain, particularly serotonin. With serotonin, it seems gut bacteria affect the brain's access to tryptophan, which is needed for the production of this neurotransmitter. It has been suggested that GABA stimulates the vagus nerve that links the gut and the brain, which then influences the brain.

In fact, research is revealing more about the influence of the gut microbiome on the brain. The finer points of this system are far from clear, but taking supplements or eating certain foods in an attempt to manipulate neurotransmitter production doesn't always achieve that result.

Some care must be taken with any attempt to manipulate brain chemistry. Eating foods reputed to be high in certain amino acids is unlikely to do harm, because nothing is made entirely of one type However, taking a supplement can be more like taking a medication, and it could do more harm than good if not done under medical supervision. Even if it's marketed as a health food, just because a pharmaceutical company doesn't produce it, doesn't mean it won't act like a medication, complete with side effects and possible impacts on other medications you might take.

Through all these challenges, amino acids do make it into the brain. There, they have to be manufactured into appropriate neurotransmitters, a process that needs a wide array of other substances to make that happen—all of which have to make it through the security cordon. Vitamins, minerals, antioxidant substances and certain fatty acids (including omega-3 oils) are all needed for this work.

Many things influence the levels of various neurotransmitters, including stress, alcohol, inadequate diet, neurotoxins, recreational and therapeutic drugs, and over the years they may contribute to problems in the brain. Only exercise and a beneficial diet have positive effects.

Nutrients for the brain

Foodworks gives you an overview of nutrients important for ageing well and reducing the risk of dementia. Before we leave brainworks, I want to alert you to nutrients with special importance to the brain and outline my suggestion of the three main ways to eat to reduce dementia risk:

> › Eat foods as close as possible to their original form—the way they came off the tree, vine or bush; out of the ground; from oceans, lakes or rivers; straight from the

paddock. That also means you minimise your intake of ultra-processed foods that are known to be potentially harmful for body and brain

> Surround your protein choice at every meal with as many different colours in vegetables, herbs, spices, nuts, seeds, grains and fruits as you can. That gives you the antioxidants and other phytochemicals to support every cell

> Add good oils to meals –olive oil and oils from nuts, seeds and oily fish containing omega-3 fatty acids.

A Mediterranean Sojourn: you are sure to have heard a lot about the Mediterranean diet and its many health benefits. That's partly because there has been, and continues to be, a lot of research on this eating style and for good reason. My three ways to reduce dementia risk here basically describe what most would understand as a Mediterranean eating plan: good protein, good oils, plenty of colours, nuts and seeds on your plate. My main alert to you moving into later age is ensuring you focus on your specific needs and make sure you get the extra protein that entails. And when it comes to protein, fish is often highlighted and intake of red meat given a negative slant. But I suggest that advice also needs to take into account what is available to you: fish and seafood sourced from pristine waterways has many benefits—the more you can enjoy the better. But if you don't know the source of the seafood you are able to buy you can't be sure how pristine were its waters of origin. If instead you can buy local, grass fed meats for the same protein that can easily be the better choice.

Omega-3 fatty acids (DHA, EPA, ALA)

Omega-3 fatty acids, DHA and EPA, are found in high concentrations in the brain and have a variety of vital roles in cognitive function (as well as in other parts of the body—namely the heart). There has been an abundance of research on DHA (from oily fish and krill), and it is accepted as a powerful protector of brain cells; but it's most likely that all the omega-3s have important roles that research has not yet completely identified, so relying on only one type may miss some benefits the others can provide. ALA (from plant sources) may help your brain cells keep up fuel supplies, and EPA (from oily fish and krill) looks like it may limit the production of βamyloid.

Vitamins B1, B2 and B3

Niacin (vitamin B3), along with the other B group vitamins (thiamine B1 and riboflavin B2) is needed in neurotransmitter production. There are a lot of claims that give niacin wonder nutrient status for the brain and, more traditionally, for heart function. Unfortunately, many of these claims are inflated. Vitamin B3 is certainly essential to brain function, and in some people is used therapeutically to assist in managing heart disease but only under strict medical supervision to avoid causing other problems. Although it's important to get enough B3, a deficiency is rare unless you have been eating poorly for quite some time, and then it will be only one of many nutrients lacking.

Folate and vitamin B12

These vitamins have distinct functions in the brain, which are covered in more detail in Foodworks, but together they assist in keeping levels of a substance called homocysteine at beneficial levels (see more in Foodworks). Both are also closely linked with brain function and deficiencies have clear cognitive impacts.

Vitamin D:

Much has been written about this vitamin in Bodyworks and we will come back to it in Foodworks. Even a marginal deficiency of vitamin D is thought to contribute to depression as well as reduced cognitive ability.

Iron

Iron is known to accumulate in the brain as we age so it's not completely surprising that such accumulation occurs in people with dementia. Researchers have been considering whether this build up might contribute to the development of dementia.

Let me be absolutely clear: iron is essential for the transport of oxygen to every cell in the brain, to make neurotransmitters and when levels in the brain are inadequate there is a link to things like ADHD, so clearly it is vital in brain health and avoiding it will cause problems.

But is iron in the brain a problem? It probably depends on what causes it, and unfortunately we don't exactly know.

One contributor may be what is left behind after a so-called microbleed in the brain. This is similar to a stroke but far smaller and hardly noticeable to those who have them. A tiny blood vessel bursts and bleeds, depriving small areas nearby of blood supply and leaving behind some iron even when the bleeding has stopped, and repairs have been done. It seems that these events individually, like TIAs, may have little effect for quite some time, especially as issues that may arise can be managed with the assistance of 'rewiring' through plasticity in healthy, active people. Over time however, they can add up until they contribute to cognitive decline and dementia.

A few years ago, media reported on studies that found accumulated iron (as well high levels of copper) in the autopsied brains of people who had Alzheimer's Disease compared to people without AD. This created some alarm and concern about eating meat and other foods that are good sources of iron.

Before you give up meat, which of course is a valuable source of protein and a range of other essential nutrients as well as iron, it looks like it is not the iron in foods that is the issue, but something goes wrong to upset the usual iron balance in the brain.

There is more risk when iron comes from supplements over the long term. Taking in extra iron without a diagnosed deficiency, even lower dose multivitamin or mineral tablets or drinks with added iron can cause you to take in more of this and other minerals that can accumulate in the same way including copper or zinc, than you would by eating reasonably well, and in forms not always as easy for the body/brain to work with. They accumulate because the brain cannot easily remove these minerals once they are in. They are needed in the right amounts, and the body is far better at taking what it needs and dealing with them when they are in food than in a synthetic form.

Too little iron can reduce cognition, but too much may have the same effect. Excess intake can come from foods, but really only if you often eat very high iron foods—liver, kidney or wild meats like venison—without also balancing those foods with plenty of vegetables, grains and other foods. If you're in doubt, speak with your dietitian or get your doctor to check your iron levels then decide what is best for you.

There is an inherited disorder called haemochromatosis (or hemochromatosis), where iron builds up in the body, potentially causing damage to many cells. People with this disorder are treated medically to reduce iron levels, usually by having blood taken regularly and may also be advised to reduce the iron they take from food, but this is not relevant for those without this disorder.

Figure 11:

Zinc, iron and copper accumulation and dementia

Research in recent years has shown that unusual accumulation of iron, copper and zinc in the brain is associated with severe problems that can lead to dementia, including accelerating accumulation of βamyloid, increasing oxidative stress, disrupting the working of the blood–brain barrier and cell death.

These mineral nutrients are also essential for all sorts of functions throughout the body and brain and deficiencies of all can be devastating.

When they come from foods, they are usually accompanied by a wide variety of other substances that assist the body to use them well, including an immense array of antioxidants. One of these is carnosine, found in many of the same foods supplying these minerals.

If, in contrast they are taken in tablet form without a diagnosed deficiency, no matter how plausible the promotional information that accompanies that product, they are far more likely to cause imbalances that the body and brain can't readily manage. What's more useful is protecting brain cells from inflammation and oxidative damage so they are better able to reduce such imbalances.

Other nutrients to check out in Foodworks are selenium, zinc, and magnesium.

The antioxidant vitamins: vitamins A, C and E

Vitamin C

Vitamin C acts directly as an antioxidant, protects vitamin E and folate from degradation and is needed to make the substances that allow brain cells to communicate and function.

Science has shown that those who have low levels of vitamin C also frequently have lower cognitive abilities.

Vitamin E

Research has found that people with low levels of vitamin

E have poorer memory and lower cognitive abilities, but unfortunately taking it as a supplement doesn't seem to boost those abilities, so the best plan remains eating food containing vitamin E.

Remember that there are many other antioxidants and other substances in plant foods called phytochemicals that are your body and brain protectors. Eating real food providing variety of colour, type and source of these is as important, probably more so, than making sure you get these vitamin antioxidants.

BRAINWORKS

PART 3

When Things Go Wrong:
How, When, What/Why?

*W*ith such a complex system where making an appropriate response to a question, managing to solve a problem or to cook and eat a meal successfully depends on finessing the activity of probably millions of separate connections between neurons, it's not surprising problems sometimes occur, and nothing short of amazing it doesn't happen more often.

Cognitive impairment and ultimately dementia is at least partly a result of damage to cells and to networks in the brain. Physical damage from head injury or a stroke is a fairly obvious issue that can have lasting impact, but it's chronic or intermittent blood flow restriction into and through the brain, and the impact of inflammation and oxidative stress, that are the long-term contributors.

A single instance of cell resources being reduced and/or toxic waste products left around brain cells longer than they should is probably of little consequence, but over decades, if those instances are repeated, the effects can add up and overwhelm the brain's usual capacity to cope.

Dementia pretenders to look out for

There are three things that can masquerade as dementia, but all can be prevented, treated or reversed. Being aware of them means avoiding a wrong diagnosis and potential irreversible damage. They are delirium, depression and vitamin B12 deficiency.

Delirium

Delirium is a serious, life threatening medical condition that can occur as a result of infection, fever, a general anaesthetic, dehydration, or from a number of illnesses.

The symptoms of delirium include confusion, agitation, disorientation, incoherent speech, unusual apathy, hallucinations and extremes of emotion, which can all occur in dementia. To a casual observer, when it looks just like dementia and there's no obvious illness or fever (usually an important clue in diagnosing delirium) it it's easy to suspect dementia as the culprit. But there is a clue: delirium usually comes on quickly and the symptoms can come and go, with a day or so in between at times, and is usually more pronounced at night. In contrast, dementia usually develops gradually over weeks, months or years, and its symptoms tend to be constant.

You'd think it would be obvious if a delirium was due to an infection or similar because there'd be pain or fever, but medication taken to control pain in other parts of the body, can mask these symptoms. Surprisingly, too, you can have infections bubbling away deep under your teeth, in your urinary tract, or even in your lungs, which cause no pain or obvious illness to alert you to their presence until they are well advanced.

It's also possible to be unaware you are dehydrated, and that too may be a potential cause of delirium. The older you get, the more likely you are to suffer delirium during an illness, particularly if you regularly take more than four different medications, have Parkinson's disease, already have dementia, or have previously had a stroke. And if it happens once, there is a high chance that it will happen again.

One thing to keep in mind is that medications themselves can cause delirium (see the list in Figure 12): you may not tolerate a new medication prescribed for you, or you might accidentally take more of one than you should. Sometimes there is an interaction between different medications, and sometimes you may have done well on a particular dosage level for many years but changes in the way your body deals with it as you age means side effects can surface, one of which can be delirium.

The take-out message is that any sudden change in your usual behaviour or of someone close to you needs a visit to the doctor. Before you even think about changing anything yourself, you must not stop taking any prescribed medication without first discussing it with your doctor, as a sudden change might itself trigger delirium or cause other health issues. If you have any concerns, organise a thorough review of your medications through your doctor or pharmacist—something that should always be done if you have experienced delirium.

Figure 12: Some medications that may trigger delirium in older age.

> **NOTE: DO NOT STOP TAKING MEDICATIONS PRESCRIBED FOR YOU WITHOUT FIRST CHECKING WITH YOUR DOCTOR. DOING SO COULD CAUSE SERIOUS HARM.**
>
> *All medications are prescribed for specific reasons and most people don't have significant problems with them or, if they do, the side effects should quickly diminish. With advancing age and increasing medical issues, problems may occur with some medications on this list. If you are concerned at all for yourself or someone you care for and especially if surgery is planned or an unexpected hospitalisation occurs, discuss your options with the doctor as soon as possible. The list is only a guide and includes common brand names. Generic brands of some medications and those released recently may not be listed here.*
>
> Medication names or types are in **bold**, common brand names in Australia are shown in *italics*.
>
> **Commonly implicated medications:**
>
> | Sedatives: | **barbiturates** (*Phenobarbitone, Amylobarbitone*) **benzodiazepines** (including *Xanax, Kalma, Valium, Serepax, Ativan, Diazepam, Rivotril, Murelax*) |
> |---|---|
> | Opioids (for strong pain): | **codeine** (marketed also as *Aspalgin, Codis, Codral, Codalgin, Mersyndol,* and in many cold and flu medications), **morphine** (*Anamorph, MS Contin, MS Mono, Kapanol*), **oxycodone** (*Endone, Oxynorm, Oxycontin*), **tramadol** (*Tramal*) and **pethidine** (*Parnate, Nardil*) |

Antihistamines:	**promethazine** (*Phenergan, Painstop syrup, Prothazine, Panquil, Seda-quell, Avomine, Tixylix*). These are older type antihistamines—the ones that tend to cause drowsiness.
Blood pressure drugs:	**nifedipine** (*Adalat, Adapine, Nifecard, Adefin*), also used for angina and Raynaud's disease; and other **dihydropyridines**.

Others suggested or that may interact with others and are worth checking:

Heart medications:	**digoxin** (*Lanoxin*), disopyramide (*Rythmodan*), **isosorbide** (*Isordil, Imdur*)
Anti-Parkinson's medications:	**levodopa** (*Madopar, Sinemet, Kinson*)
Fluid tablets:	**frusemide** (*Lasix, Urex*)
Anti-epileptic/ anti-psychotic medications:	**phenytoin** (*Dilantin*)
Some antidepressants:	**lithium** (Lithicarb, Quilonium), SSRIs (including Zoloft, Aropax, Cipramil, Lexapro, Prozac, Lovan) and TCAs (tricyclic antidepressants, including Tryptanol, Allegron, Endep, Tolerade, Tofranil)

Some NSAIDS (non-steroidal anti-inflammatories) for pain and inflammation:	incl **ibuprophen** (*Nurofen*) **naproxen** (*Naprosyn*), **diclofenac** (*Voltaren*), **celecoxib** (*Celebrex*), **meloxicam** (*Mobic*), **piroxicam** (*Feldene*), **indomethacin** (*Indocid*), **mefanamic acid** (*Ponstan*)
Some anti-ulcer drugs:	**cimetidine** (*Tagamet*)
Corticosteroid:	**Prednisone**
Some antibiotics:	**quinolones** (including *Ciproxin, Avelox, Noroxin*) **amoxycillin** (incl *Amoxil, Moxacin, Cilamox, Alphamox, Fisamox, Augmentin, Clavulin*), **flucloxacillin** (incl *Floxapen, Flucil, Staphylex*), **cephalosporins** (incl *Keflex, Ceporex, Ibilex, Ceclor, Keflor*)

Depression

Depression can look different in an older person, including more symptoms that are linked to the gut (such as bowel/stomach discomfort or changes) and sleep disturbance. It can also involve apathy, unresponsiveness and an apparent inability to communicate so it can also look like dementia. Again, if it is depression, then treatment can resolve symptoms and put you back on track.

Treating depression is vital because untreated depression causes the release of stress hormones, which can impact the smooth functioning of the brain, including creating inflammation and reducing the efficiency of making new memories.

Depression can be a part of dementia, or put you at higher risk of developing it later, so it's always worth seeking advice.

Vitamin B12 deficiency

This shares some common symptoms with dementia, is completely treatable when diagnosed early, but can cause permanent problems if ignored, so any cognitive concerns are essential to discuss with your doctor so this can be ruled out and treated if necessary. Vitamin B12 is covered in detail in Foodworks.

Blood flow impacts on the brain

Blood vessels need to be in peak health to accommodate the massive variations in blood flow that occur with changes in its activity. If they are stiffened or their capacity is restricted by inactivity and poor diet over the years, they are less able to cope with these changes. Anything that restricts flow to or through the brain or that reduces its capacity to ramp up flow as needed, even in a small way, has an impact. Complete blockage to supply quickly causes death of brain cells, as can happen in stroke and brain injury. Even the slightest restriction to blood flow, intermittently happening over many years can render brain cells less able to fuel or protect themselves causing stress that results in inflammation.

The blood also supports the glymphatic system—unless blood flows efficiently, that system can't do its clean up work either.

TIAs (transient ischaemic attacks) also known as 'mini strokes' can happen with advancing age. In these, blood flow to small areas of the brain is cut off or reduced temporarily, causing symptoms such as:

> Sudden weakness, numbness or paralysis in the face, arm(s) or leg(s)

> Difficulty speaking or understanding

> Dizziness, loss of balance or an unexplained fall

> Temporary loss of vision or sudden blurred or decreased vision in one or both eyes

> Difficulty swallowing

> Sudden severe or unusual headache.

These symptoms may disappear in a few minutes or stick around for less than a day, so it's not uncommon for them to be discounted or ignored. If nothing is done, the little bits of damage accumulate. They can also be a warning of a 'real' stroke on the horizon, and that is certainly something you want to avoid. If you get any of these symptoms, get yourself to the doctor to have them properly checked out.

Anything that contributes to changes in blood flow or to increasing your risk of stroke, such as elevated cholesterol or obesity in early or middle adulthood, needs attention for your brain's sake. Be aware that these generally need to be dealt with before you reach older age. Mid-life obesity is associated with an increased chance of dementia in later age, and high cholesterol is a significant risk factor for heart attack and stroke as well as cognitive problems—but as you already know from Bodyworks, once you're in your late 70s and beyond the situation with losing weight and even with cholesterol can be different.

Blood pressure and the brain

It's worth remembering that your brain is highly vulnerable to the effects of either high or low blood pressure. If it's consistently higher than it should be, it can damage the tiny blood vessels in the brain, starving the areas they supply of resources and even causing cell death. When blood vessels lose their elasticity, which happens as you age just like it does in your skin, it's harder for blood to move around efficiently. Unlike your skin, it's possible to keep up some elasticity in blood vessels through exercise, and the actions of muscles during activity also help blood move through them.

Low blood pressure is not as widely discussed, but in older people it can certainly present problems for the brain. One common problem is postural hypotension: that's a medical term for what happens when you stand up quickly and not enough blood gets from the body into the brain to keep it happy. Even a temporary slow down in blood flow can cause dizziness and light-headedness, easily causing a fall.

Apart from the danger of a calamitous fall, low blood pressure also means the brain isn't getting the oxygen it needs at that time, which can create permanent damage and cognitive issues over time if not addressed.

It's also vital to be aware if you have been taking medication to reduce your blood pressure for some time, that age and especially weight loss may well require a lowering of the dose you take: if that doesn't happen your medication can cause your blood pressure to fall too low and that is dangerous. Your doctor will regularly monitor your blood pressure but never forget to let them know if you have had any of these symptoms or if you have lost weight so they can consider your medication dosage.

Oxidative waste and the brain

Oxidation is the process that every one of your body cells uses to carry out its unique function, so it is essential to life. Every cell activity produces oxidative waste, which can cause damage if allowed to accumulate around that cell. Obviously this is important in your brain because its immense workload and capacity means more oxidation happens there than anywhere else.

Scientists have recently come to consider whether βamyloid accumulation could start off as part of the brain's attempt to protect itself when oxidative damage accumulates, but something goes wrong and instead of stopping when the damage is repaired, it keeps going, forming disruptive plaques that eventually affect cognitive functions.

It also seems that oxidative damage messes up the ability of brain cells to use glucose properly and disrupts the workings of the mitochondria, which are the cells' power suppliers. The process becomes self-perpetuating because mitochondria that have suffered oxidative damage start to produce more oxidative wastes, thereby adding to oxidative stress.

If damage occurs in cells of the blood-brain-barrier, in tiny blood vessels in the brain, or to glial cells then the chances of ramping up blood flow to active areas is reduced, vital nutrient access may be hampered, neurons can't achieve what they need to, and there is a much greater chance that further cell damage will occur, including the build-up of amyloid plaques and tau tangles associated with dementia. All this can happen well before any cognitive decline is evident.

It's a bit like a poorly maintained car. As the oil becomes degraded and dirty with repeated heating and cooling and extended use, and as tiny fragments of material from inside gaskets and cylinders accumulate in the engine, its efficiency reduces so it uses more fuel, blows out more smoke and generally loses power. If maintenance continues to be neglected, fuel needs may increase, wastes accumulate and things get progressively worse. Chances are it will just stop one day if this goes on long enough.

No matter what is found, however, everyone can access the protection against oxidative damage that comes from the myriad of fabulous and easily accessible substances in food that act as antioxidants— more on them very soon.

Inflammation—when the balance is upset

Inflammation is the normal response to anything the body's defence system deems harmful; designed to fight off illness and infection. It helps set up and manage any repair work that's needed and is an important part of your immune response. An 'attack' can happen anywhere in the body, so your system employs an array of communicator chemicals that gather assistance to deal with the 'invader'. These chemicals do a fabulous job when there is an active threat to be dealt with, initiating many systems and orchestrating redirection of resources as needed. If the system keeps running even though a threat has ceased, or starts up without a real threat having occurred it causes problems and that's a part of chronic inflammation.

Chronic inflammation is a bit like sitting in your car when it's stationary with the engine on and your foot on the accelerator: you are not going anywhere but you force the engine to use fuel, oil and water and to pump out exhaust needlessly. In chronic inflammation, your cells are always 'switched on'. They use resources and produce toxic waste, but with the system chronically inflamed, clean-up systems are not as effective either.

To make matters worse for the brain, inflammation causes alteration to glucose transport into the brain adding additional stress. The consequence eventually is exhaustion in some areas and the build-up of substances like βamyloid. Many researchers believe inflammation is the biggest challenge to our health as we age for these reasons, as well as because of its effects elsewhere in the body.

Why does this happen? We don't have complete answers yet, but there are many things we know play a part, and we can work with these to increase our chance of keeping it under control.

Inactivity and lack of regular exercise are big contributors. Medical research shows that a sedentary lifestyle is associated with a reduced brain volume, and that increasing the activity levels of previously sedentary people, no matter their age, reduces inflammatory activity and increases the chance of maintaining good brain function. So, exercise wins again.

Obesity is another factor and again, how that is dealt with depends on your stage in life. In early and middle adulthood obesity is a known contributor to inflammation and is thought to possibly triple your chance of developing dementia later in life. In older years, the impact of obesity is not quite the same and we need to think about it differently.

And then of course, as we have touched on here, there is the food we eat. Many foods assist in preventing or reducing chronic inflammation—on to them in just a bit.

BRAINWORKS

PART 4

Reducing Your Dementia Risk

BRAIN PROTECTION AND MORE

STAYING ACTIVE, KEEPING UP CONNECTIONS

*P*hysical activity, especially if you feel it and need to puff and sweat a bit, keeps blood flowing through the brain, reduces inflammation and more, but it also gives your brain its own beneficial 'exercise' and opportunities to develop and adapt. Working your muscles is also great for your brain.

Not surprisingly, your brain likes to learn and be challenged by new things as much as it loves being nurtured by the familiar.

Working your muscles switches on your balance systems, the senses needed to see, hear and feel as well as the resources needed to plan your activities. When you learn something you haven't done before—a new exercise program like tai chi, new card games, dance steps, sport or language, or when you make the effort to meet new people or practice skills that require concentration—your brain has to form new internal connections to keep up the pace. Combine that with keeping up with things you have always enjoyed, and you get extra benefit.

Never discount the value of keeping up social activities either. Hanging out with other people means much more to the brain than merely avoiding loneliness: it means it must continue to mastermind all the complex thought processes involved in making conversation, behaving appropriately, negotiating, and all the other aspects you need to juggle in social situations.

Interestingly, social connectedness, along with vigorous exercise, also helps keep the levels of brain derived neurotrophic factor (BNDF) up, which is probably why it's the people who combine both who tend to have the best brain health. The added bonus of remaining socially involved, from a food point of view, is that doing things socially often includes meals or, at the very least, snacks!

Resting, switching off and sleeping—all just as important as being active!

It's great to know all that time we spend sleeping is actually doing us more good than we might have thought because that's a time for our bodies and brains to rejuvenate and in the brain's case it is when the glymphatic system really swings into action.

The brain can't achieve what it does—awake or asleep—without an efficient supply of oxygen, and that can be hampered by sleep apnoea. This is a condition that reduces the amount of oxygen getting into the blood and therefore to the brain due to breathing stopping intermittently during sleep. It's usually associated with snoring and has recently been linked with development of cognitive impairment and dementia. Sleep apnoea is more common in people who are overweight or obese, and in those who smoke or snore.

Interestingly, the glymphatic system is thought to work best when you are sleeping on your side so stick to that position if it's your usual, and use strategies to avoid sleeping on your back if that is your preference.

Along with sleep, short periods of 'thought fasting' also offer benefits, a bit like the benefits that short eating fasts provide to younger bodies. This means letting the brain switch off for short periods of time while you are awake—through meditation if that's your thing, or through anything that allows it to quieten, like sitting in a park contemplating the view, spending time gazing at clouds or the ocean, fishing a quiet stream, raking leaves or sweeping, tending a garden patch, even washing dishes—anything that allows you to focus peacefully on one simple thing.

People who have lived long lives, maintaining healthy brains, are known to have engaged in some sort of meditative practice regularly within physically active daily lives. As our lives become filled with gadgets and devices designed to supply us with constant information and entertainment, it's increasingly important to find ways to give our brains a break now and then—including both good sleep and some switch off time.

Bodyweight and brain health

The impact of bodyweight on dementia risk differs depending on your current stage of life as I have said many times—sorry but it's so important!

At any age people who remain physically active, engaged in life and do good, regular exercise also have the best cognition— that is the undercurrent in everything that follows.

With bodyweight the divide for cognitive health is the same as outlined in Bodyworks: you need to do everything you can to stay lean—within the usual healthy weight range—when you're young, in early or in middle adulthood. Being leaner gives you advantages, helping keep inflammation down and supporting brain function and capacity into later life.

However, things change as you move into your 70s and beyond. Among older people and their wide range of shapes and sizes, it's those who are a bit heavier who seem to have an advantage (as already discussed in Bodyworks). They tend to have better brain function and live longer than those who are thinner. The BMI range of 22 to 27 discussed in Bodyworks also applies for the brain (as opposed to 19-25 for younger adults). That doesn't mean you can be overweight when younger and expect your brain to get off scot-free.

You might think that eating more calories than you use up just results in overweight or obesity and that's most of the story, but there is a bit more to the picture that ends up impacting cognition. The fact is that getting just a bit more energy from food than the body needs, day in, day out (called chronic overnutrition and often resulting in little or no weight gain) adds to body fat stores but more importantly can create oxidative stress and inflammation in the brain. And here's where it gets interesting—both oxidative stress and inflammation directly affect cognition, but they can also cause disruption in the energy regulation systems in the brain. That can trigger messages of hunger or a need to eat when it's not really necessary; which leads to overnutrition and weight gain, in turn increasing oxidative stress and inflammation, so the cycle continues...

For the health of your brain, anyone in younger or middle age needs to watch their long-term weight gain and if you are obese or overweight, do all you can to lose excess weight before you get to later age. Once there, aim to avoid being sedentary, get all the physical activity you can to reduce inflammation and don't pursue weight loss.

In 2020, some of the popular weight-reduction eating plans focus on periods of fasting (I've mentioned these in Bodyworks) and aim to not only cause weight loss but also reduce chronic inflammation.

Something many younger people and even well-meaning health professionals fail to remember is that most people now beyond their late 70s, even if they currently carry extra weight today, rarely did a few decades ago. If you look at images of groups of people in their 20s, 30s and 40s from before the 1960s, they were much leaner than similar images would show of 20, 30 or 40 year olds today.

Not only that but they had the advantage of living lives that were rarely sedentary and eating very few processed foods in their early lives. Recent research has demonstrated that a higher consumption of ultra-processed foods is associated with a lot of health negatives in the long term, including frailty and inflammation.

So what makes a bit of extra padding at 70+ not such a bad thing for your brain? There are a few things: body fat does more than just sit on your hips or belly being annoying—fat cells produce small amounts of some hormones, including one called leptin that helps regulate cognitive processes (as well as food intake, bone formation and body temperature) and is important in memory, learning and plasticity. There are also tiny amounts of oestrogens (estrogens) produced, thought to be of help in cognition when most other hormones are no longer circulating.

There's also the fact that cuddliness is more than just body fat, it's also muscle, bone and body fluid. Lose weight and you lose some of all of those, which can lead to problems as you now know so well.

Why eating is so important for your brain

It may seem improbable, but the day may arrive when your appetite will not constantly persuade you to make the most of every morsel that comes your way. Appetite is discussed in detail in Healthworks, but it needs a quick mention here because you must not allow it to rob you of the nutrients your brain needs.

Your appetite can make mistakes and if you allow it to convince you that you don't need to eat as much now you are older, that it's OK to skip meals or that a few mouthfuls make up an adequate meal, you can put your brain at risk. You are still running an adult sized body and brain, so unless you keep up the nutrients it needs it cannot keep you going and or keep itself protected from the effects of ageing.

It's vital to not get into the habit of missing meals or thinking you don't need as much as you once did because that can be the start of a slippery slope into malnutrition, which clearly will not help your brain. Keep eating to keep those reminders up—and if you are finding that a challenge in any way, head to Healthworks for more.

Eating to minimise oxidative damage

Antioxidant substances in food mop up oxidative wastes, so they don't get the chance to damage vulnerable cells. It makes sense that the more you can get, the better protected your brain (and your body) is.

There are hundreds of different antioxidants including some vitamins (A, C and E) and the mineral selenium, but there are many more in a variety of foods (*see* **figure 13**). Conveniently most happen to impart colour in natural foods and every different colour is down to a different antioxidant or a combination of them. The best way to make sure you get what you need is to have as many different colours on your plate at every meal. Read more on these in Foodworks, but be aware that these are best eaten in the foods that naturally contain them so you get the benefit of other substances in those foods as well.

One group of antioxidants, collectively known as the phenols (phenolic compounds), which includes many intensely coloured and flavoured foods often touted as 'brain foods' in marketing like berries, dark chocolate, turmeric, coffee and extra virgin olive oil, seem to boost production of BDNF.

It's important to always mix these up. No antioxidant works alone; they are sociable little fellows and when a mix is available, they can combine to give maximum benefit.

Figure 13

Phytochemicals and Antioxidants in foods.	
Antioxidant and/or phytochemical	**Source**
Lycopene and similar carotenoids	all yellow/orange/red vegetables and fruits, and products made from them (including jam, marmalade), tomatoes and all tomato products, watermelon

Antioxidant and/or phytochemical	Source
Lutein, zeaxanthin (also carotenoids)	kale, spinach and similar darker leafy greens, yellow-orange vegetables and fruit incl. sweetcorn, egg yolks, pink-fleshed fish and seafood (e.g. salmon and prawns), seaweed
Flavonoids	green and black tea, coffee (but not instant coffee), wine, grapes, apples, onions and berries, most fruits, vegetables and seaweed
Anthocyanins	red and purple fruits and vegetables including berries, red grapes and red wine, plums, eggplant skin, cherries, red lettuce or other vegetables with red or purple colour, raw cocoa powder and dark chocolate
Catechins	apples, cocoa, white and green tea
Curcumin (turmeric)	yellow spice in many Indian, Asian and Middle Eastern dishes and mustards
Various polyphenols	coffee, green and black tea, strawberries, raspberries, apples, whole grains, onions, garlic, ginger, mushrooms, flax seed, sesame seeds, lentils, soybeans

Antioxidant and/or phytochemical	Source
Lignans and saponins	whole oil seeds (but not the oil)—flax, sesame, seaweed, whole grains, pulses, peanuts, oats
Uridine	tomatoes, brewer's yeast, broccoli, liver, molasses and nuts
Choline	egg yolk, meats and fish, whole grains
Carnosine	animal muscle, higher in more active muscles: grass-fed and wild meats will have more. All red, white and game meats. Lower amounts in seafood but fish contains a similar beneficial substance
Resveratrol	red grape skins and red wine, blueberries, peanuts, pistachios, cocoa, dark chocolate
Vitamin A	all yellow and orange vegetables and fruits as well as eggs, butter, milk, cheese and liver
Vitamin C	citrus fruits, berries, mango, capsicums, potatoes, cabbage, spinach and Asian greens
Vitamin E	wheatgerm (in wholemeal and wholegrain bread and cereals), vegetable oils, nuts, eggs, seeds, fish and avocado

Antioxidant and/or phytochemical	Source
Selenium	nuts (especially Brazil nuts), fish, seafood, liver, kidney, red meat, chicken, eggs, mushrooms and grains
Zinc	lean red meat, liver, kidney, chicken, seafood (especially oysters), milk, whole grains, legumes and nuts.

Eating to minimise inflammation

When it comes to eating to prevent inflammation, conveniently those same foods high in antioxidants are also anti-inflammatory, so pile up the colours on your plate at every opportunity.

Some, including flavonoids and resveratrol, have antioxidant effects in your body but also move across the blood-brain-barrier where they perform important neuroprotective and anti-inflammatory roles.

A number of foods also supply substances known to reduce inflammation and protect cells, including:

> Oily fish for its omega-3 fats

> Plant-based omega-3s from walnuts, flax seeds and flax seed oil, canola oil

> Nuts, seeds, olives and avocados for their monoun-saturated fats and fibre

> Beans and legumes for their fibre and other important substances.

Oils that have undergone the least steps in production, such as extra virgin olive oil, contain antioxidants as well as protective compounds that may be removed if further refined.

It's worth mentioning that, like most things, your body deals with omega-3 fatty acids more easily when they come from food. They are beneficial substances, but when taken in amounts beyond what would usually be easy to eat (in fish oil tablets or similar), there are other considerations. Part of their action increases oxidation in cells—that's a good thing but it will result in extra oxidative waste, so it's important that if you take an omega-3 supplement you get plenty of variety of antioxidants to counter any extra oxidative wastes.

"eat foods that remain as close as possible to the way they came out of the ground, off the tree, bush or vine, out of the paddock or from the water"

I summarise all the advice on anti-inflammatory eating in the statement above. There is increasing evidence that changes made to foods during commercial processing such as repeated heating, combining numerous ingredients not naturally present in the original food, addition of sugars, fats (especially saturated), salt, preservatives or other additives can contribute to inflammation—each instance may be insignificant in itself, but ultimately they add up. Deep-fried or baked foods that are high in salt or sugar, including many takeaway foods, are likely culprits too.

That doesn't mean you should never enter a supermarket or eat fast food again—for most of us supermarkets provide a convenient, accessible source of nutritious food. However, whenever possible stick to the fresh foods—vegetables, fruits, meat, fish, dairy, nuts, seeds and legumes, along with good oils.

ADDITIONAL PROTECTION AND SUPPORT:
THE GUT MICROBIOME

There is increasing understanding that what is inside your gastrointestinal tract (your gut) has a powerful influence on your mood, behaviour and the health of your brain.

There are an almost unimaginable one hundred trillion or so (that's 10^{14} if you're a maths buff) bacteria living in the gut: outnumbering body cells and so many they are now thought of as another body organ—the gut microbiome. These many and varied bacteria are indispensable to us because they are able to harvest energy and nutrients that are otherwise unavailable from food we eat. But they do so much more than that, including producing an array of chemical messengers that communicate with and influence the chemistry of the brain.

These chemical messengers work in a number of ways: some affect the body hormone system; so can influence appetite, mood, emotion and reaction to stress. Some affect the production of neurotransmitters including serotonin and GABA (both associated more with positive emotions and calmness than with stress and aggression). It has recently been found that some also help promote brain health by nurturing the glia. What's really interesting is that if the different types of bacteria in the gut reduces (that is, there is reduced diversity), it may increase inflammation, cognitive decline and frailty as well as obesity, because under those conditions substances called cytokines that increase inflammation are produced.

Good bacteria versus bad: how a healthy gut microbiome influences the brain

You will probably have heard discussion of 'good' versus 'bad' bacteria in the gut, and it's quite true that the overall health of the gut matches the types of bacteria that live there. Diversity is probably most important because when the variety of bacteria in the gut reduces, it seems that the good ones go missing—increasing diversity means encouraging more good guys and discouraging the baddies.

The food you eat has a strong influence on this diversity: fibrous foods like pulses, wholegrains, vegetables, nuts, seeds and fruits encourage more good bacteria and increased diversity, while low fibre foods and those that have undergone more processing do the opposite.

It's not only food that has influence, the health of the brain and the health of the gut microbiome are inextricably linked through a communication hub called the gut-brain axis.

The gut-brain axis influences, and is influenced by, the emotional and cognitive centres of the brain, and this is where the system can be helpful or not. The brain affects the survival of different bacteria by changing things like the 'leakiness' of the gut wall (that allows some substances to pass between it and the blood while others are excluded) and the rate at which contents are moved along. It also releases chemical messengers and creates a local environment that helps some bacteria thrive and causes others to decline. A number of things, including a calm outlook and good stress management strategies, swing the balance towards the good guys, while anxiety and elevated stress levels give the not-so-good guys a better chance.

If the balance in the microbiome is in favour of the good guys, the messages going back to the brain tend to be helpful—promoting better mood, reduced anxiety and reduced inflammation, and as a result supporting better brain health. So, it's not only what we eat but also anything we do to manage stress that helps our gut and thus our brains.

Ongoing inflammation and unmanaged stress can also worsen a 'leaky gut', triggering autoimmune problems and worsening chronic inflammation as well as further impacting emotions and anxiety, creating a damaging cycle. The answer to avoiding this situation lies in eating food and managing anxiety and stress to help increase diversity in the microbiome, so a helpful cycle can be established

How the brain influences the gut and its inhabitants

The gut and brain are directly linked by the vagus nerve running between them, which manages swallowing, digestion and more. When anxiety and mental stress levels are low digestion settles, the heart rate calms, predominantly good things like improved memory, immune function and sleep are facilitated, while low anxiety levels are maintained. At the same time chronic inflammation tends to reduce.

A healthy gut microbiome (with a high proportion of good bacteria) aids and abets this tendency.

In contrast, heightened anxiety tends to cause the opposite and things like heart palpitations and gastrointestinal distress become more common, as well as increased inflammation and an overstimulated immune response. It's not clear which is cause and which effect, but the gut microbiome in such situations tends to be less diverse, containing fewer good bacteria and more bad.

An extra benefit of a healthy gut microbiome is that it increases the levels of BDNF, so assists in brain plasticity.

Food for a healthy gut microbiome

When it comes to food you can do a lot to boost the good bacteria and deter the bad. There are three ways to do this.

First, encourage the growth of the good bacteria already in the gut by providing nutrients that they particularly like: the fibrous so-called pre-biotic foods listed below in figure 14,which nourish and promote growth of good bacteria.

Second, introduce new good bacteria by taking probiotics or eating probiotic foods that contain beneficial bacteria. These are foods containing beneficial bacteria—fermented foods and others containing live bacteria listed in **figure 14** below.

And last, minimise foods that are thought to swing the balance of bacteria towards the bad guys: these tend to be foods that have undergone significant processing and contain high amounts of cooking fats (think battered and fried foods, commercial biscuits, cookies, commercial cakes, pies, pastries and desserts, most fast foods, fries and snack foods like chips, soft drinks and confectionery).

The thing about both pre- and probiotics is they can't do harm and often provide all sorts of other useful nutrients as well, so they are definitely worth a try. Take care if you don't usually eat a lot of pre-biotic foods though, because the fibre and other substances in them can create a lot of wind! If you want to eat more of them, or start adding new things, do so gradually and build up—that gives the good bacteria in your gut a chance to get used to the change and gradually build up and help you out.

If you already have issues with bloating and abdominal pain then get advice from a dietitian before adding any of these because they are likely to make things worse.

When it comes to probiotics and probiotic foods, different companies producing these use different mixes of bacteria and some products are more palatable than others; remember these contain live bacteria and will often require refrigeration.

There are many other strategies being developed and a lot of research going on to find the best way to achieve a healthy gut microbiome beyond using pre- and probiotics. This is likely to be different for different people and might even involve a scary concept known as faecal (or fecal) transplant. That's where gut bacteria are removed from a healthy gut, or those from a less healthy gut are 'cleaned' to end up with a high number of 'good' bacteria that are then reintroduced to swing the balance towards the good. As they say, 'watch this space'—this is something you will hear a lot about in the next few years.

Figure 14: Eating for a healthy gut microbiome

Pre-biotics:	
Grain foods:	wheat, oats, barley and rye, and foods made from them including bread, crackers, pasta, gnocchi, couscous

Vegetables:	chicory root (this is the root of the plant often called witlof—the leaves are not high in pre-biotics), garlic, onion, leek, spring onion, shallots, asparagus, beetroot, fennel bulb, green peas, snow peas, sweetcorn, savoy cabbage, Jerusalem artichoke
Legumes:	kidney beans, lentils, chick peas, all dried beans
Fruit:	white peaches, nectarines, watermelon, persimmon, custard apples, tamarillo, grapefruit, pomegranate (including seeds), dried fruit (especially dates and figs), green or under-ripe bananas (there isn't much in ripe bananas)
Nuts/seeds:	pistachios, cashews

Probiotics:

Commercial preparations with 'good bacteria' (tablets or powders)

Fermented foods:	yoghurt with live bacteria Kimchi*, sauerkraut*
	Naturally fermented pickles* (you need to look for these or make them yourself—they don't need to add vinegar because acids develop during the fermentation, so if that's an ingredient, it's probably not naturally fermented)

lassi (fermented milk drink), kefir and similar drinks

tempeh*(fermented soybean curd), miso

good sourdough bread is made using a fermentation process—it will be chewy and have the traditional sour taste if it's genuine but the bacteria themselves may not survive cooking

many traditional cheeses are fermented—Roquefort, mozzarella, Swiss, washed rind styles, gouda, traditional cheddar. It's hard to know if bacteria survive to end up in your meal, especially when heated. Interestingly, while not bacteria, the mould used to make blue cheeses may provide its own health benefits. Few, if any, processed cheeses or commercial varieties contain probiotics (those containing live bacteria may be so labelled).

*these foods are both pre- and probiotic

*these foods are both pre- and probiotic

What about nutrients or mixed supplements to boost memory or brain function?

Unfortunately, most pills and potions promoted as being able to boost your memory and save you from dementia fail to live up to their claims. You could spend a lot of money and they'd probably do little better than you could do by eating well and following the suggestions already given here.

We don't really know what causes dementia, so it's hard to develop a medication that might prevent it, but there is work underway all over the world trying to do just that. So far, nothing does as well as exercise and a varied diet. However, companies worldwide are developing products to try and prevent cognitive decline, or to reduce its rate of progress. In 2020 there are three such products on the market *Souvenaid*™, *Axona*™ and *Cerefolin NAC*™, although not all are available in all countries. In Australia, *Souvenaid*™ is distributed and its manufacturers claim it slows progress of mild to moderate Alzheimer's disease. It contains a specific combination of many of the same nutrients and substances (mostly antioxidants) discussed as being vital to the brain, in a more concentrated form.

Should you rush out and buy one of these not inexpensive products (costs vary but can be over $120 a month in Australia)? For those already facing cognitive decline or with early stage Alzheimer's, it certainly can't hurt to give it a try. The bonus when you get these nutrients in natural foods, albeit in lower amounts, is that you also get protein and other nutrients as part of the bargain, but if you are struggling to eat enough food to get these important nutrients this is a concentrated alternative. Do your research and ask your doctor and dietitian.

BRAINWORKS

PART 5

Life with Cognitive Decline and Dementia

MOST PEOPLE *DO NOT* LIVE WITH DEMENTIA: A FEW FACTS AND IDEAS

*I*t's important to remember that, while dementia is a distressing illness that naturally you are keen to avoid, the majority of people, no matter how advanced in age, *do not* develop dementia. Figures vary worldwide but in 2020 around 10% of people over 65 live with a diagnosis of dementia: of course that's worrying, but it means 90% of people over 65 *are not* living with dementia. As age increases, the number increase but still the majority do not have dementia: around 30% over 85 years—leaving 70% free of that diagnosis.

Your genes may play a part in your chance of developing dementia, but as researchers often say, 'genes load the gun but environment pulls the trigger'. Even if you have the genes that increase your risk, your life experience, including what you eat can keep your finger off the trigger: there is always something you can do to help reduce your risk.

How we live and what we eat provides support and protection needed for all players in this highly complex and sensitive system to work seamlessly.

I'm not going to give you an overview of different types of dementia or of dire statistics, there are plenty of places to find them elsewhere (there are links and references at the end of the book if you'd like more on that), but I will offer a brief look at what dementia is and isn't. We will dive more into food and activity for dementia risk reduction and brain protection soon.

Dementia? Memory lapse? Cognitive decline?

Before you write off lapses in memory as dementia or Alzheimer's, be aware that poor memory, periods of confusion or even altered behaviour do not always mean dementia has set in or is imminent. There is a lot you can do to help your brain if you're experiencing these problems. First and foremost, don't delay in discussing any concerns with your GP or geriatrician.

It's understandable to be anxious about receiving a diagnosis you don't want, but memory lapses and confusion can also be caused by completely treatable conditions. If you put off mentioning these concerns to your doctor you could miss your chance of having something treatable dealt with quickly before it causes permanent damage. And, if that visit to the doctor does deliver a diagnosis of dementia, treatments that may be able to slow its progress tend to be more effective if taken early; so don't ignore your concerns.

Increasing forgetfulness doesn't necessarily mean dementia. Everyone has occasions when they can't remember where they left the car keys or why they walked into a room. It's when you don't recall that you have a car that it could be time for concern!

Forgetfulness might even be a blessing: after all, if you

remembered every person you met and every tiny thing that happened to you in your life, it could drive you crazy.

A little beyond forgetfulness is what is called cognitive decline or mild cognitive impairment. The word cognition covers all the 'thinking' processes of the brain: coordinating things like memory, language (both understanding and speaking it), insight and judgement, problem solving and decision-making. Cognitive decline can be annoying, but it doesn't overly interfere with your everyday life. It might show up on tests and be obvious to you and to others who know you well, but it's usually manageable and doesn't always progress further. If you do regular exercise—both physical and mental—and eat appropriately it can even improve.

Unfortunately, mild cognitive decline for up to 20% of people will move on to dementia in time.

How does dementia or Alzheimer's disease differ from cognitive decline?

Dementia (including Alzheimer's disease, which is the most common type affecting around 70% of those with dementia) is not a normal part of the ageing process, and cognitive decline is only part of the picture. There are a number of types of dementia with basic differences in how they affect people but all have something in common: all interfere with your everyday life and, therefore, the lives of those around you.

People living with dementia might experience any or all of the following:

> Not being able to learn or remember new information

> Repeating stories and questions over and over

> Having difficulty finding words for familiar things

> Jumbling words and phrases

> Losing or hiding possessions

> Forgetting how or when to do everyday activities

> Making irrational or unusually poor financial decisions

> Becoming agitated and confused and even suffering hallucinations

> Forgetting things more than now and then that would usually be remembered

> Struggling to find words or names for well-known people and things

> Consistently misplacing everyday things

> Losing your train of thought or the conversation thread repeatedly

> Finding it difficult to follow the plot in movies or books

> Feeling overwhelmed by making decisions

> Making increasingly poor judgements in all sorts of situations.

While dementia is a progressive, and at this stage fatal, illness, a diagnosis by no means implies that life is over there and then, as so many people fear. On average, people have 10 to 14 years following diagnosis (though some will have five years and some up to 20). Having a good understanding of the disease, good management strategies including continued access to good food and activity, combined with sensible planning for dealing with progression of the illness means there is no reason why people with dementia cannot continue to live well for most of those years.

One thing that is far too often overlooked is a person's weight loss. Many people lose weight in the months and years before a diagnosis is made, and many continue to do so following it. This is not useful weight loss intentionally designed to shed body fat; it's malnutrition—and it has the power to snatch away quality of life, to further damage cognition and hamper physical health.

Getting a basic understanding of the way dementia might be affecting the normal working of the brain can make living with and understanding it just a bit less challenging. Without this understanding, it can be very hard not to take things personally if you live with someone who seems to be doing things just to make your life more difficult or behaving in ways they never have before. If you are living with dementia in its early stages yourself, it can help make sense of some of the things you are experiencing.

Think for a moment of the complexities involved in answering the simple question, 'Would you like tea or coffee?' That sound needs to be directed to the right place in the brain, interpreted there to give it meaning and context, then an appropriate response needs to be concocted by weaving in memories, feelings and thirst levels; then muscles need to be instructed to make the right combination of sounds at the appropriate volume and tone to relay all that in order to finally get the drink.

If there is a hiccup in any of those steps, things go awry. If the response to the question is accidentally 'Where is the car?' or if the person gets up and wanders off it doesn't necessarily mean they wouldn't like a cup of tea, it could be the connections have been jumbled. Too often people go hungry or thirsty for just those reasons.

Many people who have lived full lives and managed complex problems at work before their diagnosis are able to cover up issues for quite some time. That's partly due to a larger cognitive reserve, but also, they may be able to bring in other strategies to 'connect the dots', which might explain why some people, when diagnosed, are actually more progressed in the disease than others.

As dementia progresses more connections are lost, eventually neurons die and with that progressively increasing damage goes ability.

A person living with dementia, especially in the earlier stages when they are mostly functioning as usual and problems may not be obvious to people who don't know them well, probably gets more frustrated than an observer in situations where this confusion of messaging is happening; so patience and empathy are always important.

Does being underweight lead to dementia or dementia lead to being underweight?

It might seem logical that weight loss in dementia or in the lead up to it is caused by not eating enough food. And it can be part of the picture, but is not the complete answer. In fact, more food can be eaten or the amount going in remains the same as usual but there is obvious weight loss. We now know that dementia seems to cause the body to expend more energy than is usual so extra food is needed just to stay the same weight.

This is an intriguing finding and it probably explains why many people have already lost weight by the time other symptoms have become obvious enough to result in a diagnosis. It has always been known that unexplained weight loss can be a sign that things are awry and can herald undiagnosed physical illness like cancer, but it's now clear that it could also be a sign of cognitive decline.

For bodyweight to reduce without food intake going down, there has to be a change in one or all of the three ways that energy is expended in the body—an increase in basal metabolic rate (BMR), an increase in the energy used to maintain body temperature or extra physical activity.

If you ask most people what is the biggest contributor to energy expenditure in the body they would say exercise—it seems logical and it's so obvious when you sweat and pant and get hot that something is going on in the body, but while it certainly has a significant impact during activity, it's the basal metabolic rate that actually uses more energy most of the time.

The BMR is the energy used up doing all the things needed to keep us alive; to keep cells and organs functioning, the heart beating, the lungs pumping and significantly to keep that energy-hungry brain working. Most of the time BMR accounts for around ¾ of the energy the body uses.

A lot of energy is expended to keep the temperature of the body just right. Sweating to cool down and shivering to warm up both use more energy than you might imagine.

The extra energy used when you exercise can be huge but it's not usually that making the difference in the lead up to or following diagnosis of dementia.

It is probably a combination of all three: a slightly higher BMR, problems with temperature regulation using more than usual to keep things on track and a component of increased activity levels in some people. The latter is not usually extra gym workouts, but the combined effect of things like fidgeting, pacing, being disinclined to sit still, wandering and repetitive behaviours.

Whatever the reason, everything possible that can be done to stop weight loss progressing further needs to be done.

SO YOU LIVE WITH A DEMENTIA DIAGNOSIS: NOW WHAT?

The power of support—especially food—in dementia

I am immensely frustrated that food and nutrition is often the last thing thought of or mentioned when you sit across the desk from the doctor or specialist who delivers a diagnosis of dementia. After all, in the face of all the instructions you might receive, it is one thing that can actually be of help! Sure, it can't change the diagnosis or 'cure' anyone, but it can continue to bring joy and pleasure, and getting it right can make the difference between living life as well as possible and declining into physical incapacity and worsening health.

Importantly, providing food that nourishes the body and soul gives those offering love and support to someone with dementia something to do that can actually help.

A diagnosis certainly throws up some challenges but in no way does it mean that people will immediately cease to enjoy food as much as they always have. Some types of dementia progress quite rapidly but many do not. Connections between some parts of the brain might not be working as well as they once did, meaning the ability to communicate likes and dislikes (especially in a socially acceptable manner), or to get a meal get down safely might have gone astray. By and large these things can all be managed with a bit of creative thinking, empathy and by considering the individual.

One thing that is always true: *every person living with dementia is different!*

There is no plan that will work for all, and different types of dementia may necessitate completely different strategies. I'm not going to separate advice into different diagnoses here but offer suggestions I hope will help.

Ultimately, it's about thinking outside the box at times, always keeping in mind that everyone deserves to maintain dignity as well as enjoyment of food.

The following might happen when you present food to someone with dementia, no matter how good a cook you are:

> Straight out refusal to eat

> Lack of any response when meal is presented

> Walking away instead of sitting at the table

> Refusing to sit at the table

> Food gets pushed around the plate but doesn't make it to the mouth

> There are issues with swallowing (covered below) that mean food is spat out, spills out of the mouth during chewing or is chewed endlessly

> Food is put in a pocket, slipped under the plate or put somewhere 'for later' instead of being eaten

> Familiar foods become unrecognisable, or are perceived differently as can happen due to alterations in taste and smell.

> Cooking and/or eating utensils may not be recognised or used properly

> Frustration at not being able to communicate likes/dislikes/hunger or swallowing issues might cause food to be thrown or angrily pushed away.

The most important thing: keep people eating, minimise weight loss!

Every little thing that can be done to keep weight loss and its associated malnutrition at bay will help maintain quality of life, dignity and as much independence as possible.

Weight loss can be unavoidable in some people, especially when dementia has progressed significantly. In the later stages of dementia the combined impacts in the brain can add up until eating becomes extremely challenging and it is impossible to achieve adequate nutrition. However, for the majority of people there are many years ahead of enjoying meals and they must not be missed through complacency.

As I have said, no two people with dementia are the same, so keep that in mind as you read on—take what you think assists in your situation and leave the rest for others.

Not eating doesn't necessarily mean not hungry

This is something I am always saying in aged care and to people caring for someone with dementia in their home: don't assume that food refusal or not eating means someone is not hungry. Quite the opposite is likely to be true.

A person with dementia can feel just as hungry as always and appreciate good food as before, but as brain function and connections are impacted, being able to ask for or accept food, to express hunger or to be able to manage the complexities of food preparation or getting it from the plate and into the stomach can present huge challenges.

There are so many complexities when it comes to food. To eat it's necessary to access ingredients for meals and that could involve driving, negotiating supermarket aisles, communicating with shopkeepers, then making it home again with the items. At home, recipes must be remembered or deciphered and followed; ovens, stoves or barbecues must be managed; food needs to be plated up and cutlery negotiated to help get the final product in. It's no wonder it can get challenging to eat if the connections in the brain are messed up.

If those of us assisting someone with dementia whisk away a plate that has sat in front of them and gone cold without being touched, it doesn't mean they weren't hungry. I have seen this happen so often. I have seen people eat and enjoy meals when they are encouraged or offered an alternative, after initially saying they were not hungry.

I always advise, 'assume hunger no matter what and seek solutions'. It's about thinking outside the box, considering individual needs and working to avoid hunger and weight loss.

Some so-called 'behaviours' (a dreadful term that should be dropped but is common unfortunately) in dementia could well be signs of hunger. Many wonderful care staff on night duty offer snacks and nourishing drinks to people who pace corridors late at night to help them settle back to bed. I know if I was hungry and couldn't make you understand I wanted food or needed dignified assistance, I might just leave the table, even shout or throw things. Unfortunately, that could result in punitive action when all I might need is a good meal.

Some 'wonder diets' for dementia really just provide benefit by avoiding weight loss!

There are a lot of eating strategies or special products, often promoted on social media through heartfelt testimonials or other advertising, that people take up to try to keep dementia or its progression at bay. These can include adding coconut oil to foods and meals, making smoothies or other drinks using special ingredients or including commercial products. These, and almost all others, have a common thread in my books— they direct focus onto food and as a result end up avoiding or minimising weight loss. I'm not suggesting that some strategies don't provide benefit from antioxidants and anti-inflammatory components, but if they avoid weight loss that's probably where most of their benefit comes from.

The most important thing is ensuring someone living with dementia continues to enjoy the meals, drinks and snacks they receive, while avoiding weight loss.

If you are a carer for someone with dementia keep in mind the difference between what you need and what the person you care for needs. You may have to put aside the sorts of things you need to think about when it comes to your own diet: you might not need to avoid weight loss but you eat together.

Stick with the guidance in Bodyworks while encouraging the extras the person you care for needs.

As previously mentioned, dementia can increase the need for energy so this might be the time to embrace cream and butter and full cream milk, enjoy a bit more fat on meat, get into the fried fish and chips and use plenty of good oil and proper (not reduced fat) mayonnaise made with oil. You can look at fortifying just the portion of a meal they receive. There are suggestions for ways to boost calories and nutrients in Foodworks.

But what if someone living with dementia gains weight?

Weight gain can happen in some types of dementia and in some individuals, but it is certainly not as common as weight loss. I always encourage aiming for three things: keeping weight as stable as possible, ensuring enjoyment and quality of life is at top of mind and encouraging whatever activity gets that individual up and about.

The focus in meals needs to be good protein with as many colours on the plate as possible. If someone with dementia develops a disturbingly sweet tooth, which is quite common, there is usually little point in trying to minimise sugar because it most often leads to food being refused. It's a matter of using the sugar to carry nutrients. Fortify desserts or snacks with protein, fruits, vegetables, nuts and pulses where you can—there are some suggestions in Foodworks.

It is important to try not to restrict food. It might be hard to avoid when someone you care about starts to eat more food than usual, especially if it's what might be considered 'junk'—foods high in sugar, salt and fats—but unless they are gaining extreme amounts of weight, it's best to try to minimise the gain, certainly not to reduce weight. The fact is that eventually weight loss is likely to come into the picture with dementia progression.

My thoughts might send people well versed in the dangers of the dreaded sugar into a spin, but remember this is not 'healthy eating for all', this is guidance to allow someone living with dementia to get enjoyment from life. And the reality is, of course, this is a life-limiting illness with no known cure in 2020—eating dessert first at every meal won't change that.

Advice for carers preparing food—take heart

If you care about someone with dementia, it's very hard to not take it personally when meals and lovingly prepared dishes are rejected or worse, spat out or found later in the pot plant. Try not to see it as a reflection on your skills as a kitchen god or goddess, instead think of a way to work around the problem.

If someone wants to eat the same thing every meal or makes unusual food choices, try to work with that by adding extra nutrition to what has been chosen. There are suggestions in Foodworks that may help. Remember, if it's frustrating for you, imagine how distressing it might be for the person living with the dementia!

Tips to help good food intake in dementia

A few easy things to remember to help achieve good food intake in dementia (pick and choose what you think might help – these are not all essential for all people:

> If you are caring for someone with dementia, involved them in meal preparation if possible.

> De-clutter the table or eating space (clutter increases confusion).

> Set up an eating space that ideally is used for nothing else, or if that's not possible, set the table the same way at each mealtime.

> As often as possible keep mealtimes predictable and

routine and allow plenty of time.

> Good lighting without glare is important (the lights will most probably be brighter than you would wish— candles alone will more likely confuse things, especially if they flicker).

> TV is usually a negative distraction while quiet background music can be helpful— experiment with music to find something that helps in your situation

> Set the table so there is as much differentiation between the table and the plate and between the plate and the food as possible. Use coloured plates and contrasting tablecloth (or no tablecloth is sometimes better to avoid mishaps). Most food has better contrast on a coloured plate. Avoid patterned plates as they increase confusion and food gets 'lost'.

> Avoid noisy, busy environments for meals. If you do go to a family event or a gathering where it will be noisy or distracting, don't fret over food. Accept that nothing much may be eaten, or just offer known, liked foods (often sweet things work well). One meal won't matter; you can always try for a better food intake when you are home again.

> Reduce choice in food offered and avoid asking about food preferences to reduce the need for decision making if that's an issue.

> Even if you are not planning to eat with the person who has dementia, sit down with them as they eat and have a cup of tea or something. Evidence shows most people eat far better when they have company at the table.

> ❯ Keep food expected to be hot that way and food expected to be cold that way too. This reduces confusion.

> ❯ If you need to determine preference for foods, pictures will be a great help.

> ❯ There are all sorts of modified cutlery and crockery that can help—there are places listed to find those at the end of this section.

A note about medications

You have read, or will do elsewhere in this book, about the impact of medications on appetite, vitamin status, delirium and more. All of these can reduce both enjoyment of meals and nutritional intake.

In a person living with dementia, medication reviews must be done regularly to make sure the negative impacts don't outweigh the benefits. In the early stages of dementia considering changing or ceasing any medications might be less appropriate but as the illness progresses it is essential this happen. Quality of life and especially doing everything possible to allow a person living with dementia to enjoy every mouthful of food is essential and sometimes that will mean stopping medications that may create a barrier to that.

If swallowing is an issue

Issues around swallowing food and drinks safely are covered in more detail in Healthworks, but this is a common issue in dementia that most sufferers will face at some stage.

Swallowing food is an extremely complex process involving many brain connections and muscles, and most of the process is not under our control. We consciously chew and start the swallowing process, but after that the brain takes over. Both the conscious and the subconscious parts of the swallow can be affected by dementia and that depends on what part of the brain is affected. Most people with dementia experience swallowing issues at some time, with the likelihood increasing as the illness progresses.

In people who do not have dementia, swallowing problems can also sometimes be a sign of changes in the brain that might lead to a diagnosis. It's important to have any issues checked out by a registered speech pathologist.

Swallowing problems might not be able to be communicated by someone with dementia but there are signs to look out for, including:

> Bits of food spill out of the mouth during chewing

> Chewing goes on and on but food isn't swallowed

> Food is spat out

> Food is refused

> Food is held in the mouth without being chewed or swallowed

> Food keeps being added to the mouth even though what's there hasn't gone

> There is coughing or throat clearing during or straight after eating

> You hear gurgling or a changed voice ('wet' sounding) straight after eating or drinking

> A person may report or indicate food 'getting stuck'.

Eating safely

Before someone eats or drinks, it's vital to consider two things:

> › Is the individual alert

> › Are they upright?

It's obvious when you think about it—swallowing is just not going to go well if someone is not completely alert and that is extra important in dementia when coordination may be a little out anyway.

Food and drink has a high chance of going down the wrong way if the oesophagus and airways are squished by a slumped posture. Do everything you can to sit upright, or to help someone to do that if you are assisting them.

There is no point trying to coerce food intake or worse still, spoon food into someone's mouth if their head is dropped down and they are seemingly asleep, but I have seen this attempted and it's both undignified for the recipient and dangerous.

Some medications can impact alertness so there may be a need to look at which ones someone is taking or to consider meal timing to work with each individual.

Unfortunately dementia can mess up sleep patterns so people are drowsy during the day and awake, and hungry, at night. This is hard on carers but, depending on individual situations, making foods and drinks that are safe to swallow available through the night can be a solution. In residential care, I advise staff to offer food or drinks if someone is wandering during the night. Often residents are hungry and just providing food or drink is enough to help.

It is also important to make sure that all food has been swallowed and the mouth is clear after a meal is finished. That might seem obvious, but chewing and swallowing issues, especially in dementia, can mean some food gets left behind in the mouth—including between the cheeks and teeth or under the tongue. Bits of food can be accidentally inhaled later, sometimes well after the meal is finished.

And last but certainly not least, for people living with dementia, distraction can be an issue at mealtimes. Not only does it reduce the amount eaten, but it can also increase the chance that food is not swallowed safely. Whatever situation someone with dementia eats in, it's important to make that as free from distractions as possible and set up so it is clear that a meal is about to commence. Both help encourage good food intake and safety.

Texture modification—the good, the bad

One strategy that is initiated when there are difficulties with swallowing is that liquids can be thickened and the texture of foods modified (more on this in Healthworks). In dementia these changes can introduce additional challenges.

Foods and drinks with changed texture might not be recognised, or be refused because of their different mouth feel. Carers can help identify and describe texture-modified meals to help someone living with dementia try foods that don't look as they might be expected to.

If food or drink is refused because it doesn't look right, then thinking outside that box is needed to try and encourage intake. If that doesn't work, malnutrition and/or dehydration become greater risks than food going down the wrong way and texture modification needs to be reconsidered.

Home cooks as well as cooks and chefs in aged-care homes can have an immense impact in this: there are some suggestions on improving the appeal of texture-modified foods in Healthworks.

Dementia impacts sense of taste and smell

Changes in the senses of taste and smell in some people without a dementia diagnosis are considered to be possible signs of cognitive changes that might lead to dementia. That doesn't mean everyone who experiences change will develop dementia, but it is definitely something to have investigated if it happens to you.

Dementia itself can also impact both these senses. This can reduce the appeal of foods that might have been enjoyed previously and the experience of seeing a food then the taste not achieving what is expected can certainly diminish the amount someone feels inclined to eat.

If the sense taste is altered, foods once loved can be rejected or unusual taste combinations—even the consumption of things not usually eaten—can occur.

A problem to be aware of is that a reduced sense of smell (and taste) can mean food that is off is not recognised as such, potentially causing food poisoning.

Other effects of dementia

There are other situations that might crop up for someone living with dementia—many are not common but are worth knowing about.

Wanting to eat the same thing all the time or refusing

foods usually enjoyed

Either or both of these can occur but they just take flexibility and that 'outside the box' thinking. If food choice is monotonous it doesn't really matter as long as you can find a way to get nutrients in—adding a commercial protein powder with added vitamins and minerals into a recipe can help if it's a cooked food or a drink but consulting a dietitian would be worthwhile if it's a long-term problem.

Food stockpiling or hoarding

This is not uncommon and could possibly be a sign of hunger. The problem with it, apart from issues around food being stuffed behind the couch or in the bedside table drawer, is that the food rarely gets eaten and if it does it might be off by the time that happens. The only way to really avoid this is to 'supervise' at mealtimes.

If you are aware of the hiding place then it might work to allow food to be hidden so you can surreptitiously remove it later.

It is worth considering putting locks on food cupboards if this becomes a significant non-mealtime issue. Ideally, these should be locks that are not visible (the sort used to keep toddlers out of cupboards work well) to avoid them becoming a challenge to be dealt with or a source of suspicion. A good idea is to leave one or two cupboards able to be opened with things you would like to see eaten. You could even put a sandwich cut into quarters or other snacks like cubes of cheese or dried fruits in there—you will have to replace them of course but they just might get eaten and if they do get added to the stockpile, as long as you know where that is, you can gather it up later.

Remember, if it is a sign of hunger the best idea is to do all you can to get enough in to relieve that.

Food safety

If someone is living independently with dementia one thing those who care about that person can do is find a way to check, or help that person to check, that the food eaten is safe. So many hospital admissions for gastrointestinal upset in people with cognitive impairment are probably a result of food poisoning and it's so important that is avoided.

Doing a check without causing upset and certainly without admonishment is a great idea. This might need to be done with the person who has dementia, or might be best done without them when they are out or engaged in something else. It might involve swapping old for new of the same food.

Paranoia about food

Another thing that happens in many people living with dementia is developing paranoia. This can relate to food and especially to a belief that someone is trying to poison them. This is very scary for the person in that situation and distressing for those who care about them.

It might be possible to guide food preparation allowing the person with dementia to do all the hands-on work so they don't feel there is an opportunity for food to have been contaminated, but that is not always enough. If the concern relates to a particular food then that can be quite easily substituted, but if it is more than that, professional help is best.

Any sort of paranoia really needs the guidance of dementia support services so accessing their advice is essential.

Eating unusual things

In the behavioural type of frontotemporal dementia (FTD), and occasionally in other dementias, it is possible that things that are not food are mistaken for food. This can be anything from mildly annoying to very dangerous depending on what has been eaten. In someone with FTD it's always worth considering this if a gastrointestinal upset occurs so that the doctor or hospital might have an idea what they are dealing with.

The best plan is to organise cupboard locks as suggested above for those who stockpile or hoard food to secure dangerous substances like dishwasher power and tablets, bleach and other cleaners, nail polish and removers, paints and nasty things in the shed or garage. Go around your house if this is an issue and check cupboards and drawers, you can be amazed what is there.

Work with food memory

In people with memory impairment, especially if it's short-term memory that is reduced, the ability to recognise 'new' foods can be a challenge. Food from decades earlier is much more likely to appeal, even things from childhood—think baked custard, stewed apple, stews, lambs fry, basic meat with three vegetables. These things are often far more easily recognised than a stir-fry with crunchy vegetables; a sushi roll or chia pudding, which might be completely ignored even if the person is hungry.

Thankfully some old fashioned meats like lambs fry or rabbit, or older style desserts are having a bit of a comeback, but if something like a deconstructed lemon meringue pie, or rabbit jointed and served four ways is presented instead it might be rejected because it doesn't look like the memory of that meal suggests it should.

There are so many ways eating can be impacted. Keep an open mind and if you are new to assisting a particular person living with dementia, get to know them. Ask them what they like if they are able to tell you, using pictures of food can help. Ask their family, friends, neighbours. Put yourself in their place and think up strategies to try.

Above all, take things slowly; don't be impatient. Food provides so much enjoyment in life, be sure to always keep that in mind even if the person you care about doesn't appear to appreciate their meal— they just may be unable to tell you.

Challenges with oral health

In someone living with the early stages of dementia, teeth cleaning or denture maintenance will probably continue as usual, but in time many aspects of self-care can become challenging. It may be the coordination of the steps involved in cleaning becomes difficult, or it gets forgotten, dentures are often lost or misplaced, but also as dementia progresses they may get hidden, and be impossible to find at mealtime. Of course, losing or misplacing dentures has a huge impact on the ability to eat.

Another issue is that those who are living with dementia may not register or be able to communicate pain or discomfort as they once did.

If someone has loose or painful teeth, if their mouth is dry or their dentures don't fit well, they may not be able to communicate that effectively. Instead they may refuse food, avoid things that need chewing, throw or hide food in frustration. There are all sorts of reasons for food refusal in dementia and for changes in preferences, but ensuring that oral health is not part of the problem is relatively easy. Clearly any sort of food refusal or reduced intake is a potential problem for anyone with dementia so needs consideration.

In people in the later stages of dementia too often the need for good oral care is forgotten, or is not handled very well. Encouraging tooth brushing is a good idea of course but a time will probably come when that may not be manageable. I don't know about you, but I think if someone came at me waving a toothbrush and demanding I open my mouth to have it scrubbed, I might react somewhat negatively. Oral care is incredibly important but it needs to be handled with empathy and understanding.

Brainworks:

Take home from this section:

> Physical activity is important for your brain health

> Surround protein on your plate with as many differently coloured foods as you can for brain cell protection

> Get some good oils from fish, nuts or seeds—at most meals

> Eat food in the form as close as possible to the way it started out—fewer processed foods.

HEALTHWORKS

In this section I'm going to look at a few issues of particular significance in keeping things in your body going to support your health as you get older. Some you might need to look at differently and a few that need special attention to help you live as well as possible into your late life.

We will have a look at:

> Diabetes

> Your appetite

> Oral health and swallowing

> Nutritional considerations around illness, preparation for surgery and cancer treatment

> Common bowel issues.

PART 1

Diabetes at Later Age: New Thinking is Needed

Balancing on a tightrope and juggling at the same time

*A*s you move towards your later years if you have diabetes, you need to think about your health and diabetes management in that context. Whether you have had type 1 diabetes most of your life, developed type 2 many years ago or last month, whether you are well rounded or uber lean and fit; to make the most of the years ahead it is essential that you tailor your diabetes management to take into account the changes that have and will continue to occur in your body. Some of the cornerstones of your management up to now may actually cause harm in your later years and need rethinking.

When it comes to ageing and independence, you are no different from any other older person: what you eat and do from now on—diabetes or not—can help you age well, stay independent, and let you live the life you had hoped for.

This chapter doesn't offer a complete guide to diabetes management (there are some great resources for that listed at the end of the book) and you have already read about diabetes and brain health, but it gives an insight into ways you may need to adjust. Take the suggestions here and discuss them with your doctor and diabetes team, so that together you can decide what suits your individual needs.

Before I get on to my reasoning and suggestions, a very brief overview of the types of diabetes. If you know this all too well, just skip these few paragraphs.

Type 1 diabetes, type 2 diabetes and insulin resistance

Insulin is the hormone that is in charge of keeping blood glucose levels in line in the body, and in the brain it has important roles in memory and in maintaining the health of neurons.

Cells throughout the body and the brain rely on a constant supply of glucose, carried to them in the blood. In the absence of diabetes or insulin resistance the amount of glucose in the blood at any time is under strict control and doesn't ever go higher or lower than is best for the cells.

In type 1 diabetes, the body cells that produce insulin have been completely destroyed, so an external supply, delivered by injection or a pump system, is needed. Providing insulin from outside the body means that the internal sensors that would usually register tiny fluctuations in blood glucose levels (bgls) and then signal exactly the amount of insulin release needed to keep those levels just right, are bypassed. Insulin supplied from outside the body bypasses these sensors, so balancing injected insulin with the glucose-supplying carbohydrates from food and with activity levels can be a challenge. As a result, blood glucose levels can sometimes fall too low (called hypoglycaemia or a 'hypo') and sometimes they will rise too high (called hyperglycaemia), both can cause problems for body and brain.

In type 2 diabetes, some insulin is still produced, but the supply has become inadequate and cells become resistant to the signals from the insulin that is produced, so blood glucose levels rise above what is ideal. Treatment varies: some people take medications to help with control, some eventually need insulin injections and some are able to manage with a diet and exercise regime. Everyone with type 2 experiences high blood glucose (hyperglycaemia) at times and treatment is aimed at minimising or avoiding those times but only some who take certain medications are at risk of low blood glucose (hypoglycaemia).

Insulin resistance (IR) describes the situation where there is still insulin being produced in the body but for a variety of reasons cells fail to respond to it adequately: they become resistant. It is a part of type 2 diabetes but can also occur independently. To compensate for the resistance, extra insulin (more than is normal) is often released and that is able to keep blood glucose at ideal levels. But that also means insulin levels are higher than they really should be and that can have a variety of impacts throughout the body and brain as described below.

IR is not always diagnosed during diabetes testing because that testing usually only measures blood glucose levels, which can be normal despite high blood insulin levels.

People with insulin resistance often progress to type 2 diabetes—possibly because maintaining insulin production beyond normal exhausts the system.

It is well worth remembering that type 2 diabetes is usually a progressive illness: insulin production will generally continue to decline following diagnosis. Many people feel (or worse, are made to feel by carers, health professionals and others) that worsening symptoms are their fault, but this is not the case. Some worsening of blood glucose control over the years is to be expected; it is the therapies to manage this that must adapt. Certainly what you eat and do helps a lot and can keep worsening blood glucose control at bay for many years, but for some no matter what they do, their diabetes will progress and that is not their fault.

What is common to all types however, is once diabetes develops, it needs to be managed for life. Even if lifestyle interventions remove symptoms, most health professionals wouldn't consider someone to be 'cured' because a return to an inactive lifestyle or advancing age can cause them to reappear.

Diabetes management aims to keep bgls, as much as possible, within normal levels—what someone without diabetes or IR would achieve. It is important to keep bgls down because years of elevated bgls can damage the nerves and small blood vessels in the heart, kidneys, eyes, limbs (especially the feet) and other body systems including the brain producing complications that can be devastating and ultimately fatal.

What causes diabetes?

Type 1 diabetes is an autoimmune illness; no one knows why some people suddenly develop it, but research is happening worldwide to try and find out. What we do know is there is no known impact of what you eat or do on your chances of it developing.

Type 2 diabetes and insulin resistance (IR) are not the same: while we still don't understand completely why anyone develops these types, it may be that individuals have some sort of internal tendency, genetic or other, which is built on by so called 'lifestyle' factors like physical inactivity or being overweight. Type 2 diabetes can certainly occur in people who are otherwise fit, lean and active but both are more likely to occur in people who lead inactive lives and/or are overweight, especially in early and middle adulthood. In these years, a lifestyle change combining increased activity with weight loss can result in symptoms diminishing markedly, even disappearing altogether.

Obesity can be a sign of hidden insulin resistance because insulin plays a part in increasing body fat stores, so higher insulin production can contribute to excess weight gain, creating a vicious cycle of weight gain and worsening insulin resistance in younger and middle aged adults.

Getting back to the introduction to this section: for people in their later years, the development of diabetes and its treatment is not the same as for those who are younger.

The impact of muscle loss on diabetes

Active muscle has the ability to use glucose from the blood without insulin being required, so can reduce the demand for insulin in the body. That's a big advantage because it also reduces the chance of diabetes developing and for people who do have it, makes maintaining blood glucose levels in a healthy range easier to achieve.

It also means if you lose muscle as you age, your chances of a diagnosis in the years ahead increase and your symptoms will most likely worsen if you already have it. In fact, if people live long enough without actively working to maintain or boost their body muscle levels, most will potentially enter diabetes diagnosis territory.

This is unfortunately forgotten too often when someone with diabetes is told to lose weight in later years. You now know weight loss without exercise causes loss of body muscle, and therefore has significant consequences for diabetes.

Developing diabetes at later age

It is possible, but rare, for type 1 diabetes to develop in older adults, so when I speak of diabetes in the rest of this section, I am referring to type 2. Insulin resistance can be present, diagnosed or not, as part of that.

Once you reach your 80s, there is an increased chance of developing diabetes because age seems to challenge the body's ability to maintain an adequate insulin supply, which then combines with reduced body muscle levels.

There is significant discussion worldwide about whether diabetes diagnosed at advanced age should be treated medically at all. That's because treatment aimed at keeping blood glucose levels in control can result in reduced food intake, weight loss and other issues, impacting wider quality of life. Also, most medical treatment of diabetes aims to avoid complications that develop over decades and the fact is that is less relevant in someone who is closer to the end of their days.

Every situation is different of course but always ask if you think suggested therapy is over enthusiastic.

Managing your diabetes *and* ageing well: can you do both?

You can, but you must consider your management in a different way: ageing successfully and managing your diabetes don't line up as well as they did when you were younger. I've mentioned the aims of therapy in reducing the chances you'll develop so-called diabetes complications over the years and the need to consider the years towards the end of life differently. If you are in your 60s, 50s or younger, you have many years ahead to consider so avoiding diabetes complications is of higher importance.

For those who are older, while it is still relevant, some of the strategies used to achieve the control needed to minimise those risks can be counterproductive when it comes to getting the best from the years ahead.

I'm sure you will agree, that to live well in those years you need to avoid falling and suffering a fracture or other serious injury. I have seen far too many people permanently incapacitated by such accidents, which can easily result from over-enthusiastic diabetes management that tries to keep bgls in a tight range but doesn't account for the march of time.

Another thing that can be part of diabetes management is dealing with overweight or obesity. Many people with type 2 diabetes struggle to keep their weight down. There is no doubt that exercise and weight loss is beneficial when younger, and exercise continues to be important no matter how old you are. Diabetes or not, the same applies to weight loss in later years as you have already read: weight loss by dieting means losing muscle too. This affects diabetes control and carries all the associated health negatives you've read about in previous chapters.

It's not possible to give individual advice to each and every reader, but the following suggestions apply to many older people living with diabetes. If you are not sure what's appropriate for you, discuss what you read here with your doctor or diabetes team.

Tight control and hypoglycaemia

In younger people with diabetes, management relies on tight glucose control: aiming to keep bgls within the range those without diabetes would experience.

Australian recommendations for the population as a whole currently suggest bgls should be 4-8mmol/l (72-144mg/dl) before meals for those with type 1 and 6-8mmol/l (108-144mg/dl) for those with type 2. Two hours after meals the aim is for below 10mmol/l in type 1 and 6-10 mmol/l (108-180mg/dl) in type 2. These are similar to those in New Zealand, the United States and many other countries. That equates to an HbA1c (a test result familiar to most with diabetes and commonly used in international circles to assess diabetes control) of below 7.

These targets are necessary to reduce the chance that elevated blood glucose levels will cause diabetes complications and tight control is the undisputed cornerstone of treatment when you are younger, but tight control carries a risk that your blood glucose levels may fall below the target range, causing a 'hypo' . For a younger person the experience of a hypo is distressing but not usually dangerous. In later years it can be very dangerous.

A hypo hampers your brain's ability to coordinate body functions and increases the likelihood of a fall—a potential disaster to your health and independence at later age. If you are frail, a hypo can lead to stroke or a heart attack and experiencing frequent hypos may contribute to cognitive problems and will certainly reduce your confidence and ability to enjoy life.

It's not that I am suggesting having high bgls is a great idea, it's just that the lows can cause the life you had hoped for ahead, to be snatched away, so there has to be a different focus.

Your chances of having a hypo in later age increase for three main reasons:

1. Your ability to realise that your blood glucose levels are falling can fade because you become less able to recognise the signs before it's too late.

2. If you've had diabetes for some years a hypo can happen at a higher blood glucose level than it once did. So while 4 mmol/l (72 mg/dl) might have been your red light zone before, it could be 5 (90 mg/dl) or even higher now.

3. And then there's what you eat. Reduced appetite and eating less than you need to can have big consequences in diabetes. If you don't eat enough food—especially carbohydrates to keep blood glucose supplies up—then a hypo is on the cards.

Not everyone with diabetes is at risk of a hypo. People with type 2 diabetes controlled by diet alone or taking many oral medications are not at risk. You are at risk if you have type 1 diabetes or if you have type 2 and are either injecting insulin or taking certain oral medications which 'push' your body to make extra insulin or assist insulin in other ways. If you are not sure, ask your doctor.

Even without a hypo risk, maintaining tight control means you might sometimes limit the food you eat whether you notice you're doing it or not. That makes it difficult to get the protein and other nutrients you need to face the challenges of age. A few years of not getting quite enough protein and other nutrients can affect your muscles, bones and brain surprisingly quickly.

Relaxing diabetes control—Who? What? Why?

Relaxing your diabetes control or not is an individual decision, and you must keep revisiting your requirements every year or so, more often if you have been unwell or move beyond your 70s.

Relaxing control means allowing blood glucose levels to be a bit higher than previously, which means avoiding the chance they will fall low enough to cause a hypo—as a consequence they will also rise higher than you (and your doctor) may have been comfortable with in the past.

If you aim to avoid blood glucose levels falling below 6 mmol (108 mg/dl) then at times they are going to hit 15 or 16 mmol (270–288mg/dl) and occasionally go higher. The upper levels would have been enough to elicit an audible gasp from your diabetes team in the past, but from now on they may be essential for you.

Relaxed control has big advantages for some. It allows greater flexibility in what you eat, helps keep your appetite up if it's failing, lets you eat as well as you need to help your body confront the challenges of age, and, most importantly, greatly reduces your chances of a hypo.

However, relaxing control is not for everyone. If you are still in your 60s or 70s and quite well, then you have decades ahead and the benefits of tight control can easily outweigh the risks of a hypo. As long as you eat according to the advice elsewhere in this book, you'll enjoy those years. You'll just need to regularly reassess how you are doing as you move into your 80s and beyond, and possibly rethink employing tight control as time goes on.

Never forget that exercise plays an important part, no matter your age. Being active and getting good resistance exercise slows the progression and assists in management of your diabetes as well as all the other benefits to body and brain I keep going on about. You just need to discuss strategies for avoiding hypos with your diabetes team before you start anything new.

The following are some time of life suggestions to keep in mind around your management goals:

If you are mostly well and have had diabetes since before your 60s

Whether you have type 1 or type 2 diabetes, it may be quite a while since you were diagnosed and you still have many years ahead. If you have developed complications, they will affect your management but they shouldn't stop you remaining active and eating in the way you've read about in this book. To avoid any complications worsening and to reduce the chance of new problems cropping up, you should continue with the diabetes management strategies you already have in place, but do review these strategies as you advance in age or if you become unwell.

If you have had type 2 for many years, then you need to consider the progress of your diabetes. Even if your control has been excellent, your blood glucose levels will gradually rise and require different management. Since diet has such an influence on these levels, it's very common to assume that the gradual worsening of your blood sugar levels is because you have been eating badly. It's not all about food though, it's about the natural progression of type 2 diabetes, your body muscle reserve and your activity levels; and it might require changes in medical management. You may need to start medication, change your dose or the type you take. If you just make changes to your diet to compensate, you are likely to eat less food and get less of the nutrients you need—something you just can't afford to do.

If diabetes has only been part of your picture since your early 60s and you are not yet in your 80s

If you are active and otherwise in good health, the same applies to you as to someone diagnosed some years ago: tight control is important as long as you remain active, eat well and don't lose weight without appropriate exercise. If you are not active and healthy, you may need a different focus. The ideal will be to do what you can to boost your activity levels and follow the eating advice elsewhere in this book. If health issues limit your ability to do that, your diabetes may need to be treated as it would for someone considerably older, because the risks associated with suffering a hypo may just be too high.

If you have been diagnosed with type 2 diabetes since your late 70s, 80s or even later

It's questionable whether the sort of diabetes that develops in older age needs medical or dietary treatment at all. Diabetes at a later age is a medical condition that is distinct from the one diagnosed in younger people, but it's often treated in the same way. The effects of the dwindling ability of your body to produce insulin, combined with reduced body muscle, means that insulin production falls with age in all people so almost anyone who lives long enough can eventually develop blood glucose levels in the diabetes range. That doesn't mean you should be treated with medication, and it certainly doesn't mean it's time to cut down on the food you eat. Well-meaning friends, family and even some health professionals may encourage you to reassess your diet, but that needs to be done with great caution: any restriction on what you eat in later age, and its consequences in weight and muscle loss, are just not worth the risks.

At a later age, it's extremely important to discuss with your doctor the risks versus the benefits of medical treatment. Higher blood glucose levels can slow healing and have other effects, especially in blood circulation. That means glucose levels may need to be managed for some people, but for others it is not significant enough to require medical treatment.

It's essential that you don't start limiting the food you eat because, let's face it, any complications that are usually headed off with tight control probably won't have time to develop significantly in the limited number of years ahead—so the benefit is debatable.

Again, the main thing worth considering is exercise: even if you are already at an advanced age or are quite frail, anything you can do will be of benefit as long as it is first cleared by your doctor.

If you have lost weight and have any type of diabetes

If you have lost weight over the past few years, that's a problem in itself. You've already read how damaging the associated muscle loss from weight loss can be, but it also affects your diabetes control. It's easy to develop a vicious cycle: weight loss results in muscle loss, which contributes to rising blood glucose levels. If you then try to eat less to bring the levels down, the situation worsens—more weight goes, and with it more muscle; the cycle continues.

This is commonly seen in hospital: a frail person with diabetes who has been trying to keep their blood glucose levels down by eating less and less eventually loses so much weight and becomes so unwell they land in hospital. There they are found to be malnourished, and well-meaning dietitians supply nutritious foods and snacks. As a result the patient's blood glucose levels skyrocket and the patient and hospital staff react with alarm. It's not the food at fault—food is the essential treatment for malnutrition. The patient's medication needs looking at and a whole new plan for diabetes control worked out.

Weight loss and pre-diabetes symptoms

Weight loss can reveal diabetes or pre-diabetes symptoms (raised blood glucose levels) in later age even in those who don't have diabetes, because of the associated loss of muscle.

What you really need to do if you have been losing weight and experiencing rising blood glucose levels is to eat more and to exercise, if you can, to stop any further loss and make up for the weight and muscle that's been lost.

Special considerations: dealing with chronic kidney disease

If your kidneys have been affected by diabetes and you have been diagnosed with chronic kidney disease (also called chronic renal disease or chronic renal failure), then at some stage you may need to reconsider your intake of protein and other nutrients (especially potassium, phosphorous and salt). Kidneys can usually process any amount of protein waste, but if they are damaged by diabetes sometimes you need to eat less protein to help them cope.

Restricting protein, of course, goes against a lot of what has been recommended elsewhere in this book for optimal health as you age, so if your kidney specialist has told you to restrict your protein intake you will need the advice of a specialist dietitian to help you plan an appropriate diet.

The best protein for someone with kidney disease is the concentrated protein that comes from animal foods: all meats, chicken and poultry, fish and seafood, eggs and dairy foods (including milk powder and whey-based powdered supplements). You will also need to add extra kilojoules from non-protein foods like cream, butter or oil, and have fried foods and pastries or special supplement drinks formulated especially for those with kidney disease to avoid losing weight. That way you won't waste the smaller amounts of protein you eat by using it up as fuel. This sort of individual advice needs to come from your dietitian otherwise you won't know if you are eating what's best for you.

Frustratingly, one of the biggest problems that people with chronic kidney disease face is muscle wasting. This happens as a consequence of chronic kidney disease and significantly cuts your chances of living independently. That means you need to exercise at the same time as eating enough protein to maintain and boost your muscles without stressing your kidneys further.

The importance of exercise and how to plan for it

Exercise is an extremely important part of diabetes management at any age, but it can trigger hypos if not adequately planned. If you're on insulin or taking one of the medications listed that can cause hypos, adding exercise can bring your blood glucose levels down low enough to cause a hypo. However, that's no reason to avoid exercise—all you need to do is add extra carbohydrate-containing snacks and drinks and, in some cases, adjust your insulin or other medication dose when you exercise. Work with your diabetes team to develop a plan that's best for you. It's clear that whether you have type 1 or type 2 diabetes, whether you are lean or overweight, exercise will improve your diabetes control and help you avoid complications and continue living the life you had hoped for.

You must always check with your doctor before you start any strenuous exercise plan, but don't become complacent: you may be able to achieve more than you think you can and all of it will help you minimise the impacts of ageing.

Diabetes and your brain

Diabetes, it seems, may contribute to the development of dementia in some people. There is a lot of research happening and to find out why this might be. It may come down to how well you have managed your diabetes over the years; it may be related to repeated hypos; it may be the way insulin affects the brain cells themselves; or it may be the combined effects of a number of other players. Whatever it is, it's important to remember that it's not as black and white as has been made out in the past: having diabetes is not a guarantee you will also get dementia.

It does seem that glucose has effects in the brain that we weren't aware of until recently. Research suggests that high levels of blood glucose (even at the high end of the normal range) may also affect the brains of people without diabetes. This is worrying, because you're not always going to know they're high until they rise enough to register as diabetes, and by then they might already have had some ill effect.

Before you panic, it is important to remember that everything already said about being active and eating to support your muscles and brain holds extra sway here. In fact, exercise is the ultimate weapon. Your muscles use up excess glucose as they work to keep blood levels under control, so activity—particularly resistance exercise—is key here too. Decreasing activity in daily life may even explain the presence of higher than ideal blood glucose levels. Exercise might not be the complete answer but it's a big contributor at the very least, and has many spin-off benefits.

And don't forget—glucose is not a bad guy. Your brain relies on it as its premium fuel source. You need just the right amount—not too little, not too much.

HEALTHWORKS

PART 2

The Blessings of a Good Appetite

Our appetite makes mistakes, if it didn't, everyone on the planet would be the ideal weight all their lives without needing willpower, and that is certainly not the case!

Older age has at least one excellent benefit—you no longer need to accept a generous helping of guilt along with every mouthful of food. You have reached a milestone that signals you will probably be told to eat more rather than less, and that savouring every mouthful will be your secret to shining from now on.

I say that not because I'm trying to make all of you pile on kilos, but because appetite makes mistakes as you get older which most often end up with me hearing, 'I'm not hungry' or 'I don't need as much now I'm older' in my clinical practice, and that worries me immensely. Nothing could be further from the truth if you want to enjoy the years ahead.

There is more than one reason for this common appetite turnaround; you've already heard about your need for more of some nutrients as you age. That's pretty difficult to achieve if your appetite is tricking you into thinking you need to eat less food!

Lies and whispers—how and why your appetite deceives you

Appetite seems so simple: you eat when you're hungry and you don't when you're not. If it was that simple then why, when I look at food, especially if it's something delicious like a creamy dessert, do I get the message, 'hungry, hungry, hungry . . . must eat!' even though I know I don't really need it? And why are there also times when I have had a perfectly adequate meal but my appetite tells me I still need ice cream, when any casual observer will realise that I don't?

In stark contrast, what I often hear from my older clients is, 'But I'm just not that hungry' or 'I'm full' after a few mouthfuls, when it is obvious that three mouthfuls is not an adequate meal. It's alarmingly common, and if these messages are believed and too little food is eaten as a result, it's potentially very dangerous, posing far greater risks to your health than the few extra kilos you might be carrying.

Your appetite is a response mechanism

For most of us, food is not only about nutrition but also about our senses, and sharing and enjoying life. And that's the way it should be. You feel hungry when a whole barrage of signals combine—from habit, from your senses of taste, smell, sight, touch and even hearing, as well as from your stomach, intestines, hormones and brain chemicals. The inconvenient truth is that changes can happen in any or all of these with age. Add the considerable effects of medications, illnesses and life events, and all too soon you get those 'not hungry' messages and skip meals or eat less than you need.

Life events especially play a significant, often unrecognised, role in your appetite. Everyone has had at least a couple of days of not feeling like eating when they were ill, but grief after the loss of someone close to you, or depression, or the stress of some sort of upheaval in your day-to-day life can also kill your appetite. As you advance in age it's dangerous to unquestioningly accept such messages as legitimate reasons not to eat. You need to eat sufficiently to keep your muscles, bones and brain up to speed, and the stakes are too high now to allow appetite mistakes to dictate how much you need.

Your appetite may need a bit of TLC to get it back on track, and that means accepting two important things:

> ❯ You need to make a conscious effort to identify and then work around appetite mistakes

> ❯ From now on, even a small amount of unintentional weight loss shows that you are probably not eating enough, no matter what your appetite tells you.

I know it's difficult, if not almost impossible, to eat when your body is telling you that you're not hungry, but the stakes are too high to let that mistake take effect.

Let's consider Jessie:

Jessie is 89 and lives in long-term care. She is a lovely lady who enjoys her life there and gets on well with the staff and her friends living in the same home. She has always had a more robust, rounded body shape though is not excessively overweight. Recently she has lost a bit of weight and her appetite has declined.

She finds some foods she used to enjoy are not as appealing, so she is starting to eat only half of her morning porridge and sometimes leaves her main meal, just moving on to dessert. She says things just don't taste as good as they did. She has asked for extra brown sugar for her porridge but staff are concerned because she wants to add a lot. They also say she has chocolates stashed away in her cupboard 'for the grandkids', but they seem to be disappearing faster than their visits might suggest it should.

When I visit Jessie she doesn't complain—she's of the era when you just didn't after all—but as we talk I discuss the importance of eating and she tells me of her concerns. She is sad she is not finding the enjoyment in food she once did and is aware she 'should be' cutting down on sugar and eating better food.

Now, I always consider other factors such as medications and life events and you will read more about the impact of medication below, but in Jessie's case these didn't seem to be playing a part. My thinking in such cases is that, at 89 you have earned your treats and there is no use trying to force food on someone or try to guilt them into eating. What I try to do is use the things that do give pleasure to 'carry' the nutrition.

If a generous sprinkle of salt allows someone to enjoy fish and chips, or if three spoons of brown sugar mean Jessie will eat a full bowl of porridge, then the benefits can outweigh the risks.

Working with the kitchen staff, who love Jessie as does everyone at the home, we devised a plan. Her porridge was fortified with extra protein and calories from added milk powder (and she was allowed to add as much brown sugar as she liked). Her desserts had fruit puree and milk powder added wherever possible to boost protein and add some antioxidants and she was offered more nutritious mid-meal snacks. I discussed this with her and she was very happy to give it a try.

She stopped losing weight, in time began to enjoy her other meals again and became much happier about life.

Sometimes it's appropriate to look beyond what might be considered 'healthy eating' for the general population and instead at what you, or someone you care about, needs to get them over a temporary appetite decline hurdle, or if it's a long term issue, to live as well as possible.

If someone's appetite has declined because of an illness or other temporary issue, everything possible needs to be done to avoid reduced food intake, weight loss and malnutrition, otherwise that person can easily be on a downward spiral from which it is impossible to escape.

Eating is habit forming, but so is not eating

When you were younger, even lengthy times of poor appetite were relatively insignificant because you could bounce back easily. In your 70s and beyond, any time your appetite is reduced for a few days it's less likely to bounce back to what it was. Unless you work around that, you'll fall into the habit of eating less, and that habit will become more and more embedded over the coming years.

Fortunately, it seems that eating itself is the cure. The process of eating, especially when it happens frequently, in a mix of small meals, snacks and treats can help bring your appetite back.

Naturally I don't want eating to make you feel ill, but you need to do what you can. Eating plan 1 in Foodworks might help at first; have something every few hours, even just a small amount, use treat foods and try to have something at least every time a snack or meal is offered. Don't forget the importance of liquids. If you don't feel up to meals, try nutritious soups, smoothies and milk drinks for their nutrients as well as their fluids.

I'm overweight. Surely not feeling like eating might mean losing some weight, and that's good, right?

No it's not; I'm saying this over and over because it's so important: if weight loss happens only as a result of eating less, then what you have lost is mostly muscle and it puts your health, mobility and independence at risk.

In your later age the only way to reduce weight without also losing valuable muscle is by following a really good exercise plan suited to your health and mobility level, along with a well-designed diet that includes plenty of protein.

The other big problem with having a low appetite is that the all-important anti-ageing protein foods like meats and fish, and meals with a good variety of colours, tend to get dropped first. If they get replaced, it's often by easier, comforting options like tea with a biscuit or toast, a piece of fruit, or smaller snacks low in nutrients.

Believe me, I get it—I love my tea and toast too! However, you need to find ways to enjoy that as well as get what you need. There are some tips and strategies in Foodworks but you can't afford to miss out on protein and all those other protectors of body and soul.

Forewarned is forearmed: understanding what influences your appetite

If your appetite is trying to thwart you, understanding what might be going on behind the scenes can help arm you to counter its offensive. There are a few things at play.

Changes in your digestive system

As you eat, the appetite centre in your brain receives messages from your stomach and the rest of the digestive system to give you that familiar feeling of fullness, and then reminds you in a few hours that it's time to eat again. This system loses its accuracy as you get older and also in response to changes due to long term chronic inflammation, resulting in the wrong messages being relayed.

The 'full' feeling that stops you eating is largely a result of signals from the stomach walls when they are stretched in specific ways by the food inside. Changes to the way your stomach walls stretch as you age cause those signals to be sent earlier than they should. As a result, you feel full before you really are, and stop eating sooner before you get the nutrition you need.

While you eat, and for some hours afterwards, food gradually moves out of your stomach into your intestines. When your stomach is nearly empty, messages are relayed to remind you it's time to eat again. This process slows down considerably with age, so instead of being reminded it's time to eat your next meal after three or four hours, it can take much longer and you may feel like just one meal is able to keep you full most of the day.

Finally, food moving through your stomach and intestines triggers a number of hormones into action, sending messages to slow eating down so that food can be digested completely at each stage. Changes in these hormones, again due to age, mean you can get messages to slow eating down sooner than you should.

Any or all of these can be at play as you age, and all mean you can be tricked into eating less than you really need.

Changes in your sense of taste and smell

As you age, you lose taste buds and your sense of smell can diminish. Both of these can also be further affected by illness, medications and some nutrient deficiencies.

We all know, or can remember times when it was easy to eat entirely for the taste and smell of something delicious, and of course that's integral to the pleasure of food. So, it's hardly surprising that you can lose enthusiasm for eating if these senses diminish. What can help is finding ways to boost the appeal of your food, or sometimes choosing to eat just because you know you need it.

If your ability to taste has diminished and food doesn't have the appeal it once did, you may well find you need more salt, sugar or other flavour enhancers (herbs, sauces, gravies, cheese sauces) to stimulate your senses. Too much salt or sugar can be unhealthy, but as you become older it may be a matter of choosing the lesser evil depending on your personal circumstances. Eating too little and losing weight poses a far greater risk to your health than extra salt or sugar might.

ENHANCING FLAVOUR IN FOOD: UMAMI, GLUTAMATE AND MSG

All tastes are the result of liquified chemicals in food acting on our taste buds, with saliva liquifying any that are not already that way.

You no doubt know we register sweet, salt, bitter and sour tastes, but there is another: umami.

Umami is mainly caused by glutamate in foods. This is in many strongly flavoured foods including cured meats (ham, salamis) marinated fish, strongly flavoured fish like anchovies, dried and semi dried tomatoes, tomato paste, parmesan and other hard, strongly flavoured cheeses, dried cheese (often used to flavour processed foods) seaweed, dried mushrooms, vegemite, soy sauce and Japanese miso.

MSG and hydrolysed vegetable protein are types of glutamate used to boost the taste of foods. Some people react poorly to glutamates and years ago, MSG got a bad name as a result. Most people do not have a glutamate intolerance.

For anyone struggling to eat because foods lack taste, glutamates can help. They add taste themselves and also can enhance salty and sweet tastes so you can get away with using less salt or sugar yet achieve the same taste.

An added bonus is that glutamate stimulates saliva production, so may help if you suffer from a dry mouth.

Medications and how they play a part

It's an unfortunate fact that every medication, no matter how therapeutically effective, will often have at least one unwanted side effect and hundreds of medications affect appetite. They may directly reduce your appetite so you just don't feel hungry at all, they can change the way food tastes, sometimes adding an off-putting metallic taint, dry out your mouth and make food less appealing and difficult to swallow, or they may cause nausea, diarrhoea or constipation, with your enthusiasm for eating becoming a casualty.

Don't rush out and flush your medications into oblivion! These side effects don't affect everyone, and if you have started taking something new, the effect may wear off after a day or two. It's worth being aware, so you know there could be a reason why your cheese on toast suddenly tastes like cardboard, or you inexplicably find yourself no longer enjoying your favourite ice cream. If this sort of problem sticks around longer than a day or so, a quick chat with your pharmacist and doctor can help sort it out. It might be possible to change the dosage or type of medication, or use something to tackle the symptoms while your illness is dealt with.

Also keep in mind that when it comes to medications, the greater the number you take, the greater chance one or a combination of those will have an effect. Even something you have been taking for years with no problems; if a new medication is added to the mix it can bring on side effects you hadn't previously experienced.

This doesn't necessarily need you to have started taking something new: advancing age and weight loss can bring on problems. As you age, your body gets less efficient at getting rid of medications after they have done their job (called clearance rate), so their side effects can last longer, become more noticeable, or become evident even though you may have been taking something for years with no problems. The clearance of many medications is also related to your muscle mass, so losing weight can mean your dosage also needs to change or side effects can start up or become more pronounced.

Problems can crop up just as easily from your over-the-counter medicines or supplements (including vitamins and minerals), the ones you don't always think to discuss with your doctor. Common cold and flu tablets/liquids are likely suspects in appetite reduction, as are many preparations containing herbs, plant extracts and vitamins, which are marketed to assist a variety of conditions including sleeping disorders, hair loss, anxiety and incontinence. Over-the-counter medication or alternative therapy, no matter how seemingly innocuous, also have the potential to create side effects by interacting with medications you've been prescribed. It's always advisable to check with the pharmacist or with your doctor when you choose something off the supplement aisle shelf.

Gastrointestinal upset (nausea, vomiting, diarrhoea) is a common problem with many medications, especially antibiotics, and reduces your enthusiasm for food. Thankfully, these sorts of issues are usually temporary. It's so important to keep eating that it's worth checking with your doctor whether there is anything you can do to reduce the likelihood of problems.

Constipation saps your appetite and is a side effect of many medications. In many countries, common over-the-counter painkillers contain codeine, which causes constipation in most people. In Australia codeine-containing medications are only available on prescription but always check what you are taking with your pharmacist if you are concerned.

The number of prescription medications that can affect appetite is so extensive it's not feasible to provide a comprehensive list here, particularly as problems often stem from the combined effect of two or more medications. The following list includes some of the most likely suspects, including many you can get without a prescription. Before you head to your doctor demanding change, first try employing strategies to re-ignite your appetite such as those listed later in this chapter in 'tips and tricks to rekindle your food love affair'. They can be enough to get you past temporary appetite and taste issues and return you to the habit of eating.

Medications that may affect appetite

This is by no means a complete list but many frequent categories include:

> Blood pressure medications, particularly the ACE inhibitors

> Statins prescribed for lowering cholesterol

> Anti-reflux medications, particularly the proton pump inhibitors

> Some antidepressants

> Some diuretics (fluid tablets)

> Antihistamines, mostly the older style but contained in many non-prescription cold and flu medications (including Demazin, Mersyndol, Dimetapp)

> Metformin (a diabetes medication)

> The opiates (including codeine, endone, morphine)

> NSAID (non steroidal anti inflammatory drugs) such as ibuprofen for pain relief.

Ask your doctor or pharmacist if you take any of these and have concerns.

Illnesses and medical procedures can affect appetite

Any time you are actively fighting illness or infection, it's normal for your appetite to decrease. In younger years that is of little consequence because recovery and return to a good appetite is usually easy. When older, you can't afford to be without food for long and recovery is not as effortless.

At later age appetite can take longer to return to what it was before an illness, if it does at all, so even though it's not always easy, you need to eat your way through illness, no matter what your appetite is telling you.

Your sense of taste and smell can be affected if you have a cold, flu or an ear infection, if you have problems with your teeth, after a stroke or head injury, or after surgery or radiation in your neck, head, ear or mouth. It's important to continue to eat if at all possible. Sometimes choosing foods with different textures will help; sometimes swapping meals for high-nutrition, high-protein drinks can get you through until your appetite returns (see Foodworks for some suggestions).

Unfortunately reduced (or loss of) sense of smell and/or taste occurs quite frequently in dementia so it's important to ensure that meals, drinks and snacks prepared for someone living with dementia look extra enticing and that, where necessary additional flavour ingredients are used. There is more on eating in dementia in Brainworks.

Nutrient deficiencies can affect appetite

Inadequate intake of vitamin B1 (thiamine) and the minerals magnesium, sodium, iron or zinc can create deficiencies that reduce appetite, and zinc is also especially important for your sense of taste. Loss of appetite often means eating less, reducing your nutrient intake further and making matters worse.

If your appetite is down, blood tests to check for deficiencies should be a priority. Always ask to have those done if there is no other explanation, so any shortfall can quickly be rectified with food and deficiency-specific supplements.

Stress, depression and grief affect appetite

Stress, including grief after losing a loved one, having a serious illness or accident, suffering anxiety over life events, or having depression can cause a loss of appetite. When these things happen, eating can seem irrelevant. You may find your appetite completely absent for a while, or one mouthful will have you feeling full. You may also feel like your throat 'closes up' or your mouth feels too dry to swallow when time to eat comes around.

It's critical to be aware that eating is the path to preserving your independence and thwarting accelerated ageing. Depression in older people not only produces a low mood and emotional changes, but also produces physical symptoms such as weight loss, insomnia or agitation. Because these are physical symptoms, depression is often mistaken for other problems and not diagnosed, and therefore not treated as it should be.

Depression is more than just short-term stress. It's not a weakness and it's not something to be ashamed about. It is an illness that needs treatment like any other illness and its effects on your appetite can send you on a downward health spiral. Many strategies can help with depression: counselling, social involvement and medications all play a part. Some medications used for depression can even boost appetite a bit, which is useful if you are really struggling to eat.

Remind yourself too about the impact of the gut/brain link (Brainworks) and try to eat foods to support your gut so it can help minimise the impact of depression.

Malnutrition results in lethargy and listlessness among other things, both of which can be common in depression so it's extra important if you or someone you care about is not eating well that they are encouraged with any foods they enjoy to try and get them eating before the situation worsens. Depression must be treated as the illness it is, always discuss options with your doctor.

Bowel issues affect appetite

We have touched on the impact of medications on constipation. It makes people uncomfortable so it doesn't always miss being treated, but it is often forgotten how much it can impact appetite. There are a lot of causes of constipation as well as medications; including digestive system problems and various illnesses or injuries; but it often comes down to not eating a large enough quantity of food, not drinking enough fluids, or not getting enough activity.

Your bowels work better when you get a good quantity of food and fluids passing through them and when the actions of muscles in your belly, hips, legs and even arms move your body whenever you are active.

Have a look at Foodworks for more ways to keep your bowels moving.

Diarrhoea, at the other end of the spectrum, also affects appetite. This can be an occasional problem causing short-term issues, but for many, particularly anyone suffering from irritable bowel syndrome, it's much more than occasional and can reduce your appetite, or mean you choose to eat less to avoid the unpleasant consequences.

Tips and tricks to rekindle your love affair with food

Now that we've dealt with what causes appetite problems, here are a few things that might help you rekindle your appetite if you are getting 'not hungry' messages:

> First and foremost, watch your weight; if it falls, then you are not eating enough.

> Recognise the 'not hungry' messages as mistakes and try to eat anyway.

> Eat by the clock if you need to; have something every two to three hours. The mere act of eating, even in small amounts, can trigger a return of appetite if it's been slipping, as long as you keep it up. Missing meals will make matters worse.

> If you haven't lost weight but have been feeling less hungry, remember you still need to have at least three 'meals' each day to keep reminding your brain that it has an eating habit.

> If you have already lost weight, you need more 'meals'—5 or 6 each day. You can have small amounts at each meal but each must contain high nutrition foods (such as in the lists in Foodworks Eating Plan 1).

> If you just can't face your usual meals, take a commercial supplement or high protein drink between meals (see recipes suggestions in Foodworks).

> Be kind to yourself: use treats to tempt your appetite between meals. You are allowed chocolate, cake, potato chips, lollies, ice cream—go for whatever you love. A few treats here and there along with more nutritious foods can remind your appetite that food is pleasurable and important.

> Above all, don't give up; keep trying.

What to do if you feel full too soon and can't finish your meals

Recognise that your capacity to eat can change but your stomach doesn't 'shrink' as old wives' tales would have you believe. You cannot possibly be full on only two spoonfuls of food. Recognise the mistake.

Of course you don't want to eat until you feel ill, or make yourself sick by eating more than you really can take, but there are a few tricks you can try:

> Have just one or two spoonfuls more than you want. They're little steps in triggering the return of your appetite.

> Have liquid meals—drinks or soups. Liquids slip more easily through the stomach so can bypass the stomach's fullness sensors. (Choose from the options in Foodworks, which are high in nutrition value.)

> Add sauce or gravy to meals to make food more liquid.

> Split meals into two or three small portions and eat them over a few hours.

> If you are really struggling, have five to six small meals each day. This often makes getting enough food easier.

> Make sure every mouthful you have is a nutritious one. If you can only get half a cup of food in at each meal, make sure it's packed with the most important nutrients for your body to regain health and independence.

> If you eat bread or a cereal-based meal make sure your bread has a protein spread or filling like cheese, meat or peanut butter.

> Choose high protein cereals or add extra full cream milk powder or a high protein supplement powder to the milk.

> Make sure you make the most of every small amount you can eat.

I don't have to tell you that tea and toast will make you feel just as full as if you had added an egg or a slice of cheese to the toast, and you know how much more benefit you'll get from the added protein. It's always been that way, but it matters even more if you are eating less than you need.

A good tip is to eat the most nutrient-dense foods on your plate first so you won't waste your precious appetite on foods that give you less nutrition. Once your appetite is back you can make amends. The foods suggested in Foodworks Eating Plan 3 will help you boost the nutritional content in every mouthful you eat, but use the following as a guide:

What to choose first when you know you can't eat much

Eat first: Meats, fish, chicken, eggs or cheese—in any form.

For vegetarians, soy foods like tofu, tempeh, nuts and seeds, soy yoghurt, foods made with textured vegetable protein, quorn or soy protein, lentils and other pulses.

Full cream milk and yoghurt, soy and other non-animal milks (preferably not low fat) and yoghurts.

Any high protein and high nutrition foods specially prepared (such as those in recipes in Foodworks).

Eat next: Vegetables, grain foods and fruit.

If you do choose bread, make sure you add a good protein spread or filling such as cheese, meat or nut butter.

If your choice is a cereal-base (porridge or breakfast cereal), add a good spoon or two of milk powder, nut or LSA mix to boost protein if you can.

The special value of treats—go on, it's okay to spoil yourself!

If your appetite is challenged, 'treat' foods can help. Even the thought of your favourite chocolate, a slurp of ice cream, a wedge of triple-cream brie, a nip of sherry, a doughnut, crispy fried fish, pork crackling, something from the patisserie, a perfect peach or couple of strawberries can get your mouth watering!

When you have absorbed a lifetime of nutrition negatives that nag at you to 'avoid eating this', 'don't have that', or 'cut down on these', you can end up thinking all the foods you love are bad for you. If your appetite is dwindling, then changing to 'please have this' and 'enjoy that' and 'yes, you can have these' can do wonders. Once a day, or at least every couple of days, allow yourself a real treat—anything you really love. You don't have to eat it all, just a taste might do. A small glass of wine, a sherry or a beer, before or with a meal if you've been used to that, can help your appetite too. Treats may not contribute many nutrients, but if they help to re-ignite your appetite then they are worth it.

Spoil yourself; indulge yourself as long as you need. Often you'll find your appetite returns. Remember the rules of eating have changed now you are older: as long as you eat the foods you need there is absolutely no reason to worry about the 'don't haves' any more.

This is the time of your life when you are allowed those lovely treats. You're only old once, so enjoy them!

HEALTHWORKS

PART 3

Relishing Every Mouthful and Eating Safely

FOOD IS NOT NUTRITION UNLESS IT MAKES IT TO
YOUR STOMACH AND BEYOND

SAFE SWALLOWING AND ORAL HEALTH.

*A*mazingly enough the importance of getting food past the lips, into the stomach and beyond is sometimes overlooked when people talk nutrition in later age. It's all very well to cook fabulous meals, to manufacture and promote whizbang nutritional supplements, to wax lyrical about the benefits of eating berries from the Andes, chia pudding or kombucha; however, no food is of any use to your body or brain if you can't or won't eat it.

Among the complex array of factors that influence whether food becomes nutrition, the work of the mouth, teeth and the interplay of more than 30 different muscles that produce a swallow are naturally paramount.

Getting food from pantry to stomach to make sure people living in assisted care environments are nourished in body and soul.

There are so many reasons why nutritious food doesn't get eaten including personal preference, religious or cultural practices or boredom with the similarity of taste. In residential aged care (long-term care) homes there are extra considerations often not teased out when the focus is just on the cooking of the food. Cooking appealing food is vital, but it is just one step and in no way guarantees good nutrition or even quality of life because it must be eaten and enjoyed to achieve both of those and there are a myriad of ways to slip up between pantry and stomach.

When I (or my aged-care dietitian colleagues) look at food in aged care I always consider how a meal, drink or snack is prepared and how it looks and tastes at that time—when it's fresh and at the correct temperature. Then I also closely follow what happens to it between the kitchen bench and the person intended to eat it. If it's going to achieve nourishment of body and soul, the right meal needs to arrive at the right destination, it needs to be at the correct temperature and it needs to end up on the plate in front of a resident looking just as good as it did when first prepared. The dining area, whether that's a dining room or the bedside, needs to be set up in the way that the residents choose and enjoy. That might include TV or music in a resident's room but rarely is a blaring TV or loud show tunes conducive to an enjoyable time eating in a dining area. The dreaded medication trolley should be nowhere in evidence and all staff should spend the time during resident mealtimes either assisting those who need it or socialising with those who enjoy that to encourage interaction and improve their dining experience. If assistance is necessary with meals, that must be offered with empathy and the utmost attention to the dignity of the person eating the meal.

My aged care dietitian colleagues and I work hard to bring all those things and many more together to try ensure food is not only beautiful, but that it gets eaten and enjoyed and to identify in order to avoid the many ways that can slip. I try to bring in everyone, at every step of the process, into an understanding of how each of them can play a part in bringing those moments of joy to each person living in assisted care.

Swallowing food safely

I am not a speech pathologist, health professionals who work with people's speech, language and swallowing capacity (see Further Reading and Resources at the end of the book), so am not going to claim to have expertise in the immensely complex workings of swallowing, but I can't talk about food becoming nutrition without some discussion around safe swallowing.

Any time you have difficulty swallowing or if you cough while you eat or drink, or straight after that, it's important to have a chat with your doctor because that could mean small (or larger) amounts of food or drink may accidentally be getting into your lungs instead of making their way safely to the stomach. Even a few drops or a tiny crumb ending up where it shouldn't, can cause a chest infection and the dangerous condition called aspiration pneumonia is a result of this issue.

Another sign there might be a problem if you are assisting someone else to eat, is a change in voice—— often becoming gurgly—during a meal or straight after eating or drinking.

These signs always warrant the guidance of a speech pathologist and in fact, any unexplained chest infection also requires their input because sometimes there are no signs that food is going down the wrong way: this is called silent aspiration and is a common cause of lung infection, including pneumonia.

One reason why swallowing problems occur is muscle loss. There are over 30 muscles involved in getting food from your mouth to your stomach and they are just as vulnerable to muscle loss as any others in the body. Even a relatively small loss of muscle strength in 'obvious' muscles (for example in the legs where a loss of strength is easy to detect) also means less apparent losses have occurred in the body overall and that includes those supporting a safe swallow.

The great news though is that exercise to boost muscle activity in the body generally can also assist someone with a weak swallow. That's thought to be partly an effect on strengthening the muscles involved in swallowing themselves, but significantly, to the strengthening of muscles in the trunk, which support people in sitting upright during eating—of invaluable benefit to food getting safely from lips to stomach.

What can I do if my mouth feels dry or I feel like I can't swallow?

As you get older you produce less saliva, and this can be exacerbated by some medications. Saliva plays an essential role in your ability to taste foods, maintain the health of your teeth and swallow smoothly. Your taste buds register the taste of foods properly when the flavour chemicals food contains are in liquid form and that needs the addition of saliva for anything that is not already a liquid.

Without the lubrication of saliva, food may feel like it's getting stuck or become difficult to get out of your mouth and down to your stomach easily.

The feeling that your throat closes up as you eat can also be caused by stress and grief, and the strategies below will help you continue to eat in these circumstances:

> Swap solid meals for nutritious drinks (recipes in Foodworks) or liquid meals such as soups or casseroles for a while.

> If problems crop up when you start a new medication, check with your doctor about making adjustments.

> There are good products on the market to help lubricate your mouth, ask your pharmacist or doctor.

> Make sure your meals have extra liquid in them or add extra sauces or gravy. Add cream, custard or ice cream to desserts.

> Stew your fruit or buy it canned in syrup or juice instead of fresh. The softer texture helps you to swallow.

> Have a drink on hand and sip it as you eat.

Medications can cause a dry mouth

Reduced saliva flow affects both the taste of food and swallowing ability and unfortunately hundreds of medications can cause that to happen. Ask your doctor if you are having problems and take any of the following types of medication:

> Antihistamines

> Antidepressants

> Diuretics (fluid tablets)

> Parkinson's medications

> Many blood pressure medications

> Asthma inhalers (rinsing your mouth after every use can help)

> Medications to stop seizures

> Antipsychotics.

When swallowing is not safe—the good and the bad of changing food texture

One strategy that a speech pathologist might recommend when there are difficulties with swallowing is that liquids are to be thickened and the texture of foods modified. To achieve this, a thickening product is added to drinks and some liquid foods to give them a texture more like honey or custard. Foods and meals may need to be cut up, minced or pureed instead of being presented as their original state. Some other foods might also be restricted because they are crumbly or dry and cause extra challenges.

People who have had experiences with food going down the wrong way are often very happy to adopt such changes to avoid that very unpleasant, often terrifying experience. But others resent or resist them.

It is quite possible to make texture modified foods appealing with just a bit of effort (there are some suggestions in **Figure 15**) and there are some good pre-made products on the market that you can keep on hand also (some are listed in 'Further Reading and Resources' at the end of the book). Unfortunately, the effort is not always applied as well as it should be and people become uninterested in the food, then eat and drink less and suffer the consequences. It's a bit more difficult to modify many of the protein foods so they hold their appeal, and that is an issue in itself if protein intake falls.

Often texture-modified foods are fortified with additional protein, kJ and nutrients to make up for reduced intake, so production of these meals requires some special attention.

Figure 15: Some tips on preparing texture-modified foods.

Texture modified food should be prepared and presented to increase its appeal no matter its texture. Unfortunately, when changes in texture first occur, its common for people to eat less of those so it is even more important to ensure texture-modified foods taste great and you do all you can to maintain joy in eating.

Suggestions include:

> Try to keep the meal experience as much the 'same as usual' as possible: the dining area and table setting needs to be appealing and any assistance offered must be provided with empathy and close attention to every individual's dignity.

> Try to make texture-modified meals look as much like those not modified as possible to trigger food memory.

> If foods are pureed, you can use food moulds to make the end result looks as much like the original food as possible.

> Put some of the food (the meat dish for example) in small ramekins or similar and arrange vegetables carefully scooped around that to remain as appealing as possible, this works well for minced texture.

> Make sure only the items that require modification are altered. Some people require meat minced but their soft vegetables don't need mincing for example.

> Do not stir the meat and vegetables together (unless it is specifically requested).

> Make sure to vary gravy or sauces added to each meal—using the same brand commercial gravy or sauce mix with every meal can make everything taste the same.

> If you are dealing with food being provided in a care home or similar, make sure that foods on the regular menu that are also safe for those on texture modification are available to everyone. This might include mousse desserts, moist puddings or desserts, thick soups, pate, soft cheeses. Just because you or a loved one needs most meals modified in texture, that may not always mean a different meal is required to what others receive.

Smelling, tasting and being enticed

Eating well is far easier to achieve when food smells and tastes good and both of these senses can be impacted by age.

Use flavour enhancers like salt, spices, sauces or even MSG (read more on this and using umami-containing foods in Foodworks). You only need a very small amount to boost flavour and 'make your mouth water'.

ORAL HEALTH

It comes as no surprise that if your teeth and your mouth aren't as healthy as they could be you are not going to be able to eat as well as you need to. What is surprising is how often that is forgotten or overlooked in care.

If you have an infection in the teeth, gums or deep below the teeth, that causes inflammation extending far from the mouth and contributes to inflammatory damage throughout the body and the brain, so prompt treatment is important for more than your oral health. It's quite possible to be unaware of the pain of an infection under a tooth if you take a pain medication for an unrelated issue , so regular dental checks should be part of your health plan and if bad breath becomes evident, that can be a sign things are not as they should be.

Of course, poor oral health, painful teeth or gums, a dry mouth or ill-fitting dentures can make eating otherwise enjoyable foods difficult, contributing to malnutrition.

One thing to consider is the influence of saliva in oral health. I've touched on this previously, but for oral health generally there are extra considerations. Saliva not only moistens food so it can be chewed properly, be tasted effectively and formed into the right consistency to be swallowed, but importantly it contains substances that help protect teeth from decay and infection. So, any time saliva production is low, teeth are at additional risk. There are hundreds of medications that can cause these problems, including recreational drugs such as marijuana (cannabis) and cocaine. Consult your pharmacist or doctor if you are having any issues.

There are also extremely important cosmetic and social aspects to teeth, oral care and dentures. For someone who usually wears dentures, not having them available or not wearing them changes the way they look significantly and for many people that is understandably challenging. Also, if someone is not keeping up oral hygiene then others might react to them negatively with resulting distress, especially if they are not aware of the reason for the problem.

Keeping up regular dental visits is important so potential problems can be dealt with. One thing many people may not consider is that your dentist needs to know what medications you are taking: some must be ceased before any dental work is done for your own safety. That includes blood-thinning medications and one of the newer ones for osteoporosis, which may need to be stopped months before any dental surgery is performed to avoid potential damage.

I want everyone to get the chance to enjoy every mouthful and that just can't happen if chewing is difficult because of teeth or denture problems, or if pain or inflammation reduces enjoyment of food previously savoured like a good steak, nuts and seeds, crunchy vegetables, crisp fruits or grainy bread.

Oral health issues go well beyond the mouth

Infections and disease in teeth, gums and supporting structures (periodontal) cause more than discomfort, pain and cosmetic issues in older people. They also contribute to:

> Inflammation throughout the body

> Poor food intake and consequent malnutrition

> Swallowing problems and aspiration pneumonia

> Blood loss and consequent anaemia.

HEALTHWORKS

PART 4

Resourcing Your Body for Surgery and Cancer Treatment

Preparing for surgery

I am constantly amazed by the lack of discussion and awareness about the extra nutrition you need before and after any surgical procedure. It makes sense when you think about it, especially what you eat in the week or so before the operation. Nutrition is so important at that time, your needs can be immense and yet are often completely overlooked.

If you are planning to have surgery of any kind, eating appropriately in the lead-up as well as afterwards will help you come out of it the best you can. As with so many other things, this becomes more important as you get older.

There is plenty of research evidence that shows inadequate nutrition in the lead up to and immediately following surgery greatly increases your chance of post-operative infection, slows recovery and leads to re-admission to hospital. Yet the benefits in minimising those risks, increasing the body's rate of repair and getting you out of hospital more quickly by ensuring great nutrition before and after any procedure are often forgotten in all that paperwork and planning before you enter the hospital doors.

Eating to boost nutrition in the lead up will help things run smoothly and have you back on your feet faster.

Surgery, or repairing damage from an accident or sudden illness places immense additional demand on your body due to the widespread trauma from injury, inflammation or infection, and you will have had no opportunity to boost your nutrition beforehand. Eating while in hospital can unfortunately be the last thing you or even the medical staff might consider, but it is absolutely essential if you plan to slot back into life where you left it. If the surgery is planned, you are at a decided advantage because you get the chance to eat to support your recovery well ahead of those extra demands.

Your body reacts to the assault of surgery by producing 'stress' hormones. These are important in helping your body cope, but cause additional muscle breakdown (remember—that's where your reserves of protein are stored). After any type of surgery you'll need many nutrients, but protein is by far the most important because you'll be using huge amounts to repair and rebuild damaged tissue, fight infection and replenish lost blood. The bigger the surgery the greater your needs will be and if you suffer infection your needs skyrocket.

Instead of being able to eat well at a time like this, you usually have to fast before the procedure then deal with a reduced appetite and limited intake afterwards. Without the protein from food, your muscle reserves have to supply what's needed and you may need three or four times the amount you would usually require, so that's an enormous drain on your muscles.

It's little wonder that the older you are, the more you may struggle to recover from surgery, but if you consciously work at eating well and doing activities beforehand to boost your muscle reserves, your recovery will be quicker and the road to your ongoing independence will be much smoother.

So what do you need to do?

First and foremost, boost the amount of protein you eat in the lead-up to your surgery and keep up whatever activity you can to support your muscles. Use the strategies for recovery from illness given in Part 1 of Foodworks, that means a protein food as the basis of three meals a day, plus an extra serve between meals.

For many people the best option is to have high protein drinks between or with meals. You can make them at home according to the recipes in Part 3 of Foodworks, or buy any of the commercial supplements. Among them are some especially formulated for surgery patients. They contain particular amino acids (the building blocks of proteins) including glutamine and arginine and other nutrients considered to be especially useful.

You need to get something that suits you as well as your budget. Some supplements are quite costly but the less expensive, more widely available choices—or those made at home—are often just as effective. The worst option is if you do nothing.

This is not a time to be concerned about the possibility of gaining weight. This higher protein diet is a short-term prevention and recovery strategy. One week of higher protein intake before your hospitalisation should be enough for minor surgery; two weeks at least would be advisable for a major operation, especially if you aren't likely to return to normal eating directly after the procedure.

If you have lost weight in the lead-up to your surgery then you may need more than that to make it up and to prepare you for what's ahead. If you have lost weight before planned surgery you should seriously consider committing extra time rebuilding your muscle before you go ahead. Of course you can't put off life-saving surgery, but heading into an elective operation with already depleted reserves is asking for trouble and may very likely hamper your recovery.

The nutrients you need to pay particular attention to, apart from protein, include:

> Zinc (wound repair)

> Iron (blood loss)

> Vitamin C (repair of damaged tissue)

> Antioxidants.

Commercial supplements contain a range of nutrients along with protein, so if you are using home made protein drinks you can add a general purpose multivitamin—but as always, check with your doctor and/or dietitian that these are appropriate for you. If you are eating well, the additional vitamins and minerals probably won't be needed. It's protein that is critical at such times.

What about emergency surgery?

In all the flurry of medical activity what you eat is too often forgotten, but exactly the same applies as if your surgery is planned. You face potentially huge losses of protein from your muscles, and if you don't eat well, that will escalate.

You can feel helpless as your medical and nursing team swing into action, but eating to aid your recovery is one thing you can take control of and do for yourself. Eat and eat well if that's possible—especially protein foods and as many colours as you can, or get supplements to boost your intake. You won't be able to stop some muscle loss, but you will be able to do a lot to slow the loss down and set yourself up for a faster recovery.

Unfortunately there isn't nearly enough focus in most hospitals on nutrition. Dietitians work hard to elevate its importance, but budget constraints and lack of awareness too often don't allow the proactive menu planning that would help your recovery. That's a pity because, quite apart from the benefit to you in recovering faster, all sorts of costs to the health system can be cut if patients eat with recuperation in mind. If you heal more quickly, savings are made in wound care, in medications, and in the length of time you need to remain in hospital.

You can help yourself no matter what food is available by making sure you eat; and if you can't face solid meals there are often high protein supplements available as alternatives—ask the food service team or the dietitian. You can also have your own supply of supplement drinks and snacks brought in by friends or family if that's acceptable to the hospital; just check with your doctor or the dietitian to be sure that what you are having is right for you.

I can't stress enough how important this is. You might have to take the initiative yourself if it's not suggested to you.

> **A side note if you are heading for weight loss surgery:**
>
> I would not usually recommend weight loss surgery for someone older because of the high likelihood of muscle loss having long-term impacts that outweigh the benefits of lost body fat. But, individual circumstances vary and people in their later 60s and beyond do undergo these procedures. For them, advice on eating in the lead up to the operation can be quite different.

It is common for surgeons to recommend extremely low kJ (calorie) intake in the weeks before the surgery in order to reduce the fat built up in the liver. This frequently involves consuming one of the very low energy supplement 'shake' products on the market. These provide minimal kJ but provide protein and other nutrients so are of assistance in preventing surgical complications and assisting in recovery in younger people but may not be adequate if you are older. I strongly suggest seeking the guidance of an accredited practicing dietitian experienced in the care of older people if you are considering this surgery.

Food to support you through cancer treatment

The following information is not about cancer prevention. My aim is to give you a focus in that confronting limbo between your diagnosis or tests and when your treatment starts.

You have to give your body all the resources it needs to support the cancer therapies ahead and at the same time ensure your chances of independence afterwards. To do that, you need to eat foods to help your body fight the cancer itself and minimise weight loss (especially muscle) so that doesn't eventually cause you further damage.

You will recall that losing enough body muscle is eventually fatal in itself, but you can do a lot to head this off before you start any treatment, as well as during the treatment phase.

There is no doubt that a never-give-up attitude is crucial in the fight; and eating right is certainly part of that strategy.

What to do right away

Right away you can start to prepare for the assault of surgery, radiotherapy, chemotherapy or a combination of these. The same strategies that prepare you for elective surgery will work here, but because you can't be sure exactly what's ahead it's worth adding a bit of extra nutritional input. You need high-protein, high kilojoule-foods, supplements and meals, and you should keep up whatever activity you can to help boost your muscles.

It's especially important to keep the variety of foods up, particularly those multi-coloured vegetables, fruits and other foods that supply antioxidants. Don't forget, it's a combination of antioxidants and other components in these complete foods that provide the benefit, not extracts alone. (To refresh your memory, there was a more complete list of antioxidants in Bodyworks)

You're going to get all sorts of advice on diets and supplements, and it's common to consider 'cleansing' diets or to take on advice to avoid meat, dairy and other specific foods. To give your body the best chance to face what may be ahead this is not the time to start cutting out foods that provide protein and other beneficial substances, many of which might be animal foods. If you feel that big diet changes will help you, then consider them only when your treatment is complete. Right now you need protein foods and their readily available nutrients like iron, zinc and vitamin B12. Focus on keeping your protein and energy up and add coloured foods for protection.

It's different if you are already vegetarian or vegan: you should already be getting the variety of colours, but you must work to get the extra protein you need from nuts, seeds, soy foods, meat alternatives and pulses. That will mean larger amounts of plant protein foods and the addition of soy or other plant-based liquid supplements if necessary.

Don't forget that boosting your muscles and fully utilising your protein intake, relies on being as active as you possibly can. If you are already fit when you are diagnosed you have an advantage. Exercising, or at least being active, is another thing you can do to boost muscle as well as help you to feel positive.

What to do while you are being treated for cancer

Nowadays cancer is frequently confounded and sent into remission as a result of advanced medical therapy and maximising the nutritional value of your food intake. However, there is no medical therapy that can stop the muscle loss that comes with cancer and that is accelerated by any reduction in activity and eating.

Some cancer treatments are going to have you struggling to do even light exercise or eat anything at all. You'll also need a lot of rest to help you recover. Take every opportunity to do whatever activity you can between rest periods, and eat good high protein foods even if it's only a few mouthfuls at a time. As soon as you feel better you can increase both.

If you can't cope with solid meals, then having a variety of high protein supplements and consuming as much as possible is a great idea. Use the suggestions in eating Plan 3 in Foodworks. Juices can be a fantastic way to get in lots of antioxidants, cancer protective substances and vitamins, but they are low in protein. Adding a neutral flavour supplement or blending in nuts or seeds will supply protein and make a drink more like a smoothie.

Beware of big claims

Beware of tablets or supplements with only one or two ingredients, no matter how good they sound. All the evidence suggests that different food components and nutrients work together better than they do individually. In large dosages, many food components, herbal preparations and even otherwise harmless substances can act completely differently to how they would if you got them from your food, and can even upset the actions of your cancer medications. You must check everything you plan to take with your doctor or cancer team to be sure you won't cause yourself more harm than good.

What to do if you are battling nausea

Nausea, whether caused by medications, illness or, ironically, by not eating will have you convinced that getting anything down is absolutely impossible. However, eating can be the way to deal with it.

Not eating can be the culprit, so you need to trick your body into getting enough to reverse this cause. The key is to take small amounts frequently and usually to start eating as soon as you wake.

Just a sip or a small bite every 10 or 15 minutes is enough. And don't let up, because everything you can get is doing you good.

Sweet drinks (sweetened with normal sugar or glucose, NOT artificially sweetened)—from the fridge or with ice—are a good choice. You can get Lucozade (a commercial glucose soft drink) or for most people lemonade is fine—straight or diluted, fizzy or allowed to go flat. Ginger helps reduce nausea and can be taken in any form, including ginger ale. Peppermint does the same, so enjoy a cup of peppermint, ginger or regular tea, and add glucose powder or sugar to this too. You can dilute these drinks with water if they taste too strong.

Many people find plain or slightly salty cracker biscuits good too, or a small handful of dry breakfast cereal. Nibble on this as soon as you get up, and about 10 or 15 minutes before meals to help reduce nausea and get more out of your meals.

Ask your doctor about your medications. If any are contributing to your nausea, there may be alternatives you can take. There are also special medications you can take before meals to help reduce nausea.

It's undeniable that eating or undertaking activity when you are nauseous, when food often just doesn't stay down and when you feel sapped of energy, is a huge challenge. No matter what your treatment includes (surgery alone, or with radio or chemotherapy), anything you can do to hold onto and boost your muscle reserves will help you.

HEALTHWORKS

PART 5

Moving Along: Managing Bowel Concerns

Constipation

*T*his is a topic for a whole book in itself, but it's such a big issue in older age it needs addressing here. It's an everyday problem for many people and is often overlooked or given inadequate attention among the many different medical problems you may face.

Dealing with constipation is really important because not only does it make you feel miserable, it also reduces your appetite, often makes you nauseous, can cause urinary incontinence and contribute to urinary tract infections.

Understanding how your digestive system works can help determine the strategies to deal most effectively with constipation.

Your bowel is a long tube, narrow in the small intestine and wider in the large intestine. Food passes along the upper part in liquid form and water is gradually absorbed as the contents move along, to produce a solid stool by the end. If food passes through the system too fast it will come out quite liquid (diarrhoea) but if it moves too slowly it becomes dry and hard and difficult to move out. There are bands of muscle surrounding the bowel that contract rhythmically to push the contents along, and they work best when there's enough bulk for them to act on. The bulk comes from eating plenty of food, especially those containing dietary fibre because this combines with water to keep the contents being not too soft and not too hard. It's a bit like squeezing a toothpaste tube: when it's full it's easy to squeeze the toothpaste out, when empty it's much harder. If your intestine is mostly empty, with only occasional hard lumps, then those lumps can be challenging for your muscles to push along, resulting in a slow and under-active system. As you get older your muscles can become less efficient, and sometimes the nerves that coordinate their activity don't work well so you don't perform as well in the bowel department as you once did.

In your abdomen, your large bowel (also called the colon) runs from your lower right side near your pelvis, up to just below your ribs, across to your left side then down to lower left where it finally becomes the rectum, where its contents are passed out.

One common result of your bowels working too slowly or inefficiently is that gases, which are normally produced during food breakdown, accumulate instead of being moved along, causing not only flatulence but also gas build-up higher in your bowel. Gas can get trapped anywhere along the colon, causing bloating and a tight, swollen and often painful abdomen. In a chain reaction, when gas builds up, the muscle bands can't work effectively and their rhythmic pulses are not able to push the gas or the solid contents along efficiently, worsening the problem. The longer the bowel contents stay inside you, the more gas gets produced and the more water is removed from the stool, making it more difficult to pass through and causing extra discomfort.

Gentle massage of the abdomen using a circular motion starting on the lower right, moving up the right side, across under the ribcage then down the left side can help move gases along and reduce this discomfort.

Dehydration and eating too little food can contribute: your appetite is reduced when you are constipated, but cutting down what you eat gives the intestinal muscles less bulk to help them do their work and dehydration contributes to drying out the stool. Staying active and getting plenty of exercise will help move gas out, reduce discomfort, and help the contents move along as well.

Faecal (fecal) impaction and overflow diarrhoea

Another thing that can happen in constipation is called overflow diarrhoea, which is a form of faecal impaction. This is a confusing and potentially devastating condition because the chance of bowel accidents happening stops people getting out and about.

What happens in overflow diarrhoea is the bowel contents move so slowly that hard and quite dry masses of faeces build up and are unable to be pushed along. They fill or block areas in the bowel so that fluid builds up behind the large mass (though not enough to cause a bowel obstruction, which is a medical emergency). All this fluid either seeps past and flows out, or gushes out suddenly. You often don't get a warning, which can be extremely distressing and embarrassing. It's also confusing, because it seems like you have diarrhoea but it's actually constipation.

This is considered to be very common among the frail elderly, especially those who are less mobile and unfortunately, because it's often thought of as diarrhoea, its treated with medications designed to reduce bowel movements, which is obviously going to make it worse. A simple x-ray can identify impaction, often revealing large areas of bowel filled with contents that are not moving along. These situations require medical management to get things back on track, but then prevention strategies will help avoid ongoing issues.

The effect of medications on constipation

The side effects of medication are often the cause of bowel issues in older age because many commonly used medications contribute to constipation. Be sure to discuss any problems you are having with your doctor or pharmacist. If you are prescribed an opioid for pain (codeine, morphine, pain patches such as Norspan and Durogesic) then you will usually need a laxative to balance its effect. In many countries, over-the-counter medications, including most cold and flu medicines and many pain relievers, contain codeine (in Australia, medications containing codeine are only available on prescription). If you are prone to constipation try to avoid these pain relievers, but if you do have to take them, be prepared for your bowels to take a few days to return to normal.

Some medications affect the action of the bowel, while others change the absorption of water from the stool. Antibiotics reduce the number of bowel bacteria and, since normally around a third of the content of the stool is bacteria, that reduces bulk and makes it more challenging to move contents along. If you have taken antibiotics, a course of probiotics when your antibiotics are finished (tablets, yoghurt or drinks containing live bacteria cultures) can rebalance essential gut bacteria and help reverse the problem.

There are many medications to treat constipation. They work in three main ways:

> Keeping liquid in the stool (stool softeners)

> Speeding up the rate that food passes thought the bowel (bowel stimulants)

> Increasing the bulk of the stool (bulking agents and fibre supplements)

> A combination of all three.

You need to work with your doctor to get the dose right, as some medications to treat constipation can go too far and cause diarrhoea.

Something else to be aware of is that iron and calcium supplements can also cause constipation—not when these vital nutrients come from food (iron, especially from meats, and calcium from dairy foods)—but when they are taken as tablets.

The good and the bad of fibre

The most common nutritional strategy for constipation is to get plenty of fibre. Fibre is a bulking agent and does two things: it absorbs water and holds it, adding bulk to the stool and keeping the bowel contents soft. Adding fibre means you also need extra liquids. Often people cut down on fluids to try to avoid having to pass urine frequently, but not getting enough fluid makes constipation more likely.

The other benefit of fibrous foods (see the list in **figure 16** below) is they encourage the growth of healthy bacteria in your bowel. Not only does this support the microbiome and its brain benefits, but a large percentage of the weight of faecal contents and the stool that is eventually passed is dead bacteria. This is normal, the bacteria have done their work and are being replaced in the gut but importantly they also bulk up the stool.

Figure 16: Dietary Fibre in Foods

High fibre foods to include daily (increase gradually if necessary):

> Wheat, oat or other cereal bran

> Psyllium husks

> High fibre breakfast cereals (usually bran based)

> Dried figs, prunes and other dried fruits

> Legumes, pulses of all sorts (including baked beans)

> Nuts and seeds

> Wholemeal/wholegrain foods and breads

> Vegetables such as cabbage, kale, root vegetables, onions, peas, corn, kohlrabi, turnips, broccoli.

There are a few problems that can crop up with fibre in older age: one is that many foods containing fibre are bulky and tend to fill you up before you get a chance to eat all the protein and other nutrients you need. And, with the exception of pulses like lentils, soybeans and the like, they contain little or no protein themselves. As you've already read, protein and antioxidants need to be your main food focus. Luckily many antioxidant foods are also fibre foods—think pulses, wholemeal and wholegrain breads, cereals and grains, fruits (especially dried), vegetables and nuts.

If you can only eat small amounts then getting enough bulky high fibre foods can be difficult, and that's where fibre supplements can help. There are a number of options: bran, psyllium and similar products can be sprinkled over cereals and meals or mixed into a smoothie. Commercial fibre powders, including the brands Benefibre and Metamucil, come flavoured or unflavoured and are mixed with water or other liquids. The benefit of the unflavoured varieties is that they can be mixed into high protein drinks, soups and juices. The very commonly prescribed Movicol is a mix of fibre with a bowel stimulant.

Fibre can reduce the absorption of some minerals, including calcium, iron and magnesium, so you need to be sure to get plenty of these if you are taking fibre supplements over the long term.

When you add extra fibre you need to give your system time to get used to the change or it may cause excess gas build-up and discomfort. Start with a small change and if you are using a fibre supplement start with as little as a teaspoon a day. Build up according to your doctor's advice or the instruction on the container until it's working, and then stick with it so the problem doesn't start up again.

It might also help to add some probiotics (foods containing beneficial bacteria that you have read about in Brainworks). Adding good bacteria can help your bowel cope with the fibre and boost the volume of your stool.

It's essential when you increase your fibre intake that you also keep your liquids up because too little fluid with a lot of fibre like bran or psyllium can dry out the stool, making matters worse.

Many people avoid drinking a lot because they don't want to make lots of trips to the toilet to wee. Remember the dangers of dehydration discussed in Brainworks and the fact that concentrated urine in the bladder irritates it, causing increased urge to go even if there is not much to pass.

If you experience gas and bloating that these strategies don't resolve, you may need to look at avoiding some very high fibre or specific foods, or at least avoid having more than one high fibre food at a time. It's not a strategy that would usually apply if you were younger, but it may be necessary to help you manage symptoms in older age.

If you have concerns, consult a dietitian to help you plan a food intake. Diet adjustments can help people with IBS (Irritable Bowel Syndrome) – read more in **Figure 17.**

Figure 17: A note on IBS (irritable bowel syndrome and pre-biotic foods)

For reasons we are only just beginning to understand and that may well involve the gut-brain axis, some people develop an 'irritable' bowel. The lining of an irritable bowel can become excessively 'leaky' and hypersensitive to components of foods that most people tolerate well. Individuals may suffer chronic diarrhoea or chronic constipation and significant abdominal pain and discomfort.

One therapy that can dramatically reduce symptoms, bringing welcome relief to those living with IBS is a scientifically researched therapeutic diet known by the acronym FODMAP. It restricts a number of foods containing substances that cause the gut bacteria to react, creating symptoms. Some of the substances restricted on this diet are pre-biotics and for people with IBS, foods containing these may not be tolerated as well as they are by others.

If you do have problems with IBS, get professional advice from an Accredited Practising Dietitian before adding a lot of extra pre-biotic foods. There is increasing evidence that probiotics can help people with IBS so planning how to add those that are tolerated is worthwhile.

There is also gathering evidence that working with the brain to reduce gut hypersensitivity in people experiencing IBS symptoms might work well. That in no way means the symptoms are 'all in your head' but recognises there is a problem in the gut that the gut-brain link might be able to assist. Psychologists engaged in this work may well be able to help.

The gut brain connection

You read in Brainworks about the connection between the brain and the gut (aka the bowel). It is clear that your gut is a highly 'emotional' organ. Stress, grief, depression and many other emotional situations affect not just your mood but how your gut functions. Emotions can cause your bowels to speed up or slow down: the former causing loose bowels or diarrhoea and the latter contributing to constipation.

It's possible that for some people with irritable bowel syndrome (IBS) this is part of the problem. I'm not going to cover IBS in detail (there are resources at the end of the book in Further Reading and Resources) but it certainly needs a mention here. Everyone with IBS is different and experiences this frustrating condition differently. There are therapies that aim to reduce IBS symptoms by focusing on the brain. That isn't because 'it's all in someone's head'—far from it! In IBS, the gut is often overly sensitive, especially to pain caused by changes in contents or to accumulated gases and other factors and it 'overreacts'. That oversensitivity is not something an individual can control directly or they have caused, but therapy that aims to calm brain activity can also reduce gut oversensitivity as well.

There is certainly a link between stress/anxiety and bowel activity: in some people stress causes bowel slowing, in some speeding up. In both of these and in IBS, working to reduce stress levels with meditative brain activity and exercise is important. Just as important is eating to support a healthy microbiome as discussed in Brainworks: improving the health of the microbiome improves brain health, which then helps bowel function.

And it always remains true that every bit of physical activity you can do will help by assisting in pushing contents along, reducing inflammation and stress and increasing the chance you will eat enough food to help your bowel out too.

Constipation is such a complex condition it's very difficult to provide a complete range of solutions here, but the following strategies summarise some things to help keep your bowels moving:

Stay active and get plenty of exercise. This is absolutely essential as the muscles in your abdomen and around your pelvis work as you exercise and as you move around and help push the bowel contents along. In fact, just taking up a good walking and activity program may be all you need to reverse worrying constipation. It's also the way to help move any accumulated gases along and out—and sure, farting may be a bit antisocial, but if you don't get those gases out they will cause pain, and you don't need that. Just pick an appropriate moment, along the same line as if a tree falls in the forest and no one hears it, did it really fall?

Eat! Your bowels need volume.

Add extra higher fibre foods or supplements if you need to.

Avoid dehydration. Not drinking enough fluids will make stools harder.

Healthworks:

Take home from this section:

> Keep reassessing medications and diabetes management as you move into later age—things may need to change

> Appetite often declines with age, but don't let it fool you—you still need to eat to keep an adult body and brain running well.

> Be prepared nutritionally before you have surgery and eat to recover afterwards

> Keep up fluid intake—dehydration causes many problems for body and brain.

FOODWORKS

PART 1

Getting What You Need From Food

I am not going to discuss every nutrient people need—there are plenty of books that cover more general nutrition advice (I've given you a couple of suggestions at the end of the book). Here, the focus is on those nutrients that have special or increased importance for you once you are looking towards, or enjoying your later years. They take into account extra wear and tear your body has encountered, inevitable changes in your digestive and other systems, illness impacts and medications you take.

Before you read on, a reminder of what to consider when thinking about vitamin tablets or supplements: forget the idea that, just because small amounts of nutrients are recommended for good health then large amounts must be even better: it's just not true and in later age intakes above what you need can cause problems.

Don't waste your money, because you can only use the vitamins and minerals immediately needed. Any extra amounts boost the sewerage system, not your body. Some things, taken in excess, can even accumulate when they shouldn't and potentially cause problems, while others can interact with your medications, disrupting the smooth running of your body systems. And anyway, Mother Nature gets the balance right when you source your vitamins and minerals from a wide variety of foods; excess intakes can set up imbalances. The other great thing about real food is it contains all sorts of other substances, many of which work alongside nutrients to help us use them efficiently. When you replace food with tablets you forego these benefits.

Having said that, if you like to take a general purpose multivitamin tablets supplying doses up to the recommended daily allowance, that's unlikely to cause harm. If you have been diagnosed with a deficiency, naturally that must be corrected with an individualised supplement but it's important that you don't pick up a bottle of two from the seemingly endless shelves of vitamin and mineral tablets in your discount pharmacy. If you do plan to start taking something, let your pharmacist or doctor know to avoid interactions with medications.

FLUIDS

Water, juice, tea or milk? What and how much to drink to ward off dehydration?

Most people should have between six and eight glasses or cups of liquid each day. What you need is about 30ml of water for every kilogram you weigh (or 1oz for every 2lb bodyweight) so you can work it out if you really want to. It doesn't all have to come from water; in fact, if you find eating three good meals a day as well as the occasional snack a challenge, drinking a lot of water can make things worse because if you're full of water you may not feel like eating, and will miss out on valuable nutrients.

You can get the fluid you need from many different sources:

all sorts of drinks—including tea, coffee, juices, milk—and many different foods including fruits, soup, desserts, jelly, casseroles—anything not dry, really.

If you are eating well and haven't unintentionally lost weight, get the liquids you need from water because you won't need the extra energy (kilojoules or calories) that juices, soft drinks, milk supply.

If you have lost some weight or are struggling to eat well, then combine nutrition and liquids: choose drinks offering extra energy and protein such as flavoured milk, protein shakes and smoothies. Choosing soups, casseroles and desserts that are moist like custards or ice cream adds to fluid intake also. If you are really struggling to eat, don't fill up on water before a meal if it means you won't feel like eating the food you need.

Usually a drink with each meal as well as something in between should give you enough fluids. Just be careful if you like to drink tea with your meals, because it can affect how well you absorb some nutrients, including iron, from your food. If you are not eating well, getting enough iron from food can be a challenge anyway, so if possible, it's best to enjoy tea between meals.

PROTEIN

You know already from Bodyworks why protein and muscle are important, so it's vital to eat to get what you need and that can be as much as an elite athlete requires as you age!

Athletes need extra protein to keep their muscles up to scratch because of the extreme activity levels they subject themselves to. You have read of the impacts of age on muscle and protein increasing requirements and that is added to if you are unwell, have an accident or surgery, and to compensate for any muscle losses. Getting enough when your needs are extra high can sometimes mean needing to fortify the foods you eat or add in a high protein drink.

Even without the stress of illness or muscle loss, and even if you feel and eat well, you have reached an age when you need to think of the amount of protein in each of your meals.

Getting enough of the right stuff

When you are well and active, getting the protein you need is usually as easy as building your meals around a good protein food and adding multi-coloured vegetables, grains and fruits— ideally at three meals a day. The exact amount you need depends on your weight and health, so giving an individual guide is not practical here. There are international guidelines on how much younger adults are advised to eat (about 0.8 to 1 gram protein per kg a person weighs) but those don't necessarily apply to those who are older. It will be a while before it is agreed on exactly what to recommend but the gathering consensus is:

For those who are mostly well, an amount around 1.2 grams of protein for every kilogram you weigh (or 0.55g per pound of weight) is often suggested as the ideal level (some researchers suggest 1.5 grams per kilogram per day—0.68g per pound). That means you might need 70 to 90 g a day, spread as evenly as possible across all meals.

Figure 18 gives you guidance on the amount you need to eat to get 20 grams of protein—work with that to plan your day's intake, always remembering there are times when you are:

> › Recovering from illness

> › Heading for surgery or have just had an operation

> Immobilised (or recently have been) due to illness

> Losing weight (and therefore muscle)

> Exercising to boost your muscle

> Moving into later old age.

At these times you may need 15 or 20 grams more protein each day, the equivalent of an extra two small chops, two eggs, four slices of wholemeal bread or two cups of lentils.

Figure 18

You might need to aim for 30g of protein per meal. These lists are designed to give you an idea of how much food you need to eat to get 10g protein. You can mix and match to make up a meal.

Eg: 2 egg omelette with 30g cheese and 1 slice of toast

Bowl of pasta with a can of tuna and tomato passata

1 small chicken breast with vegetables

2 cups of rice with at 1 cup of dahl and 1/2 cup nuts

Food	Approx percentage of this food which is protein	Amount of this food you need to eat to get around 20g protein. (Standard measuring cup, tablespoon Tbs, teaspoon – tsp)
High Protein Supplements:		
Whey protein isolate	94	22 g 2 level Tbs
Soy protein isolate	83	25g 2 1/2 level Tbs
Hemp Protein	50	40g about 4 Tbs
Nutritional yeast flakes	45	45g 4 1/2 level Tbs
Skim milk powder	35	57g about 6 Tbs

Meat, chicken, fish, lean only (cooked)	30 - 35	60g portion approx. size of a pack of cards 1 lge chicken drumstick, 2/3 small can tuna/salmon etc drained
Meat, poultry, fish, seafood with skin, fat, light crumb/ batter (cooked)	20 - 30	100g portion approx. size of 1 1/2 - 2 packs of cards
Vegetarian 'meat alternatives': quorn, veg sausages etc (cooked)	20	100g portion approx. size of 1 1/2 - 2 packs of cards
Egg	13	150g 3 X 50g eggs
Commercial milk additives - dry (eg: Milo™, Ovaltine™, Aktavite™)	12	160g about 2/3 cup when used without milk 100g about 1/2 cup when mixed with 250 ml milk
Milk, Lassi, Amasi (milk maas)	3-4	600ml (or approx. 80g/3 dessertspoons milk powder)
Yoghurt, kefir	4 - 9	400g about 2 cups/ 1 1/2 cups thick, Greek-style yoghurt 230g 1 cup kefir
Parmesan, other very hard/dry cheese	40	60 g 2 Tbs
Cheddar and other 'hard' cheeses	25-30	70 g. 3-4 commercial- sized slices, 2/3 cup grated
Cottage cheese, brie and similar 'soft' cheeses	15-20	110g. 1/2 cup
Lupin uncooked flakes Lupin cooked flakes	40 20	50g about 1/2 cup 100g about 1 cup
Hemp seeds (hulled) Hemp flour	32 20	60g about 1/2 cup 80g about 1/2 cup

Chick pea flour (gram or besan)	22	80 g about 1/2 cup
Soy beverage, soy yo-ghurt	3-4	600ml beverage or 400g yoghurt
Dried peas/beans (fava, broad beans, peas, ad-zuki, edamame peas etc)	25	80g 4 small handfuls Or fraction under 1/2 cup
Soybean cooked (Eda-mame)	18	105g slightly heaped 1/2 cup
Quorn meat substitute (uncooked)	15	130g 1 heaped cup mince style/2 fillet/1 large patty
Kidney beans (cooked)	14	140g a bit under 1 cup
Tofu, miso, bean curd	12	140g about size of 2 packs of cards
Lentils – including urad (black), puy, yellow and red Chick peas, channa, mung beans and moong dahl **(cooked)** Maize meal (cornmeal/grits/pap) raw, **dry:** **cooked:**	8-9	220g 1/2 regular can or 1 generous cup 220g 1 cup (raw) 600g 3 cups (cooked)
Green peas cooked/raw, baked beans	5	250g 1 1/4 cup
Hulled pumpkin seeds	30	70g 1/2 cup
Peanuts, peanut butter (no additives)	25	80g 2/3 cup or 3 good handfuls

Food	Protein (g)	Amount
Almond, pistachio, sunflower, sesame seeds (& tahini), wattleseeds, LSA mix	20	100g about 1 cup
Nuts/seeds: Cashew, Brazil nut, walnut, pecan, pine nuts, flaxseed (linseed), poppy, chia seeds	15	130g about 1 1/3 cup
Rice and quinoa (cooked)	3	660 g about 6 cups
Porridge (rolled oats, made with milk)	5	400g about 2 cups
Commercial breakfast cereal made with wholegrains/ labelled as higher protein	20	100g more than 1 cup depending on the variety
Bread	10	200g about 5 – 6 regular slices

If getting that amount in sounds like an impossible feat, then fortifying foods by adding protein and/or extra kJ to them or trying high protein drinks or special supplement drinks can make life easier. Boosting your protein intake as soon as you possibly can after illness or surgery will help your recovery—even if you are still laid up.

Don't always expect to see improvements in the mirror, but remember than an adequate protein intake will certainly help you regain strength and ability, as well as support your body in all those other important internal functions you read about earlier in this book.

If you are trying to regain strength and muscle then getting protein foods with plenty of essential amino acids, especially leucine, is also worthwhile. Look at figure 19 to give you some ideas on getting leucine from food.

Figure 19: amount of food to provide 2 g leucine*

FOOD/SUPPLE-MENT	QUANTITY	QUANTITY in approx. everyday measure	TOTAL PROTEIN in this serve size (g)
Whey Protein Isolate	20	2 Tbs	18
Skim milk powder	60g	6 tbs/ ½ cup	22
Beef, Poultry, Seafood	120g (raw weight)	Approx. the size of the palm of a hand	25
Eggs	3 eggs	3 eggs	19
Cheddar cheese	70g	3 commercial slices or 3 cubes 2cm^3	
Cottage Cheese	140g	½ cup packed	
Peanuts	120g	Just less than a cup	
Almonds	130g	Just less than a cup	26
Kidney beans	350g	Most of a can	23
Lentils	380g	A full can	18
Tofu	400g	block about half a brick size	48
Whole milk	600ml		22
Soy beverage	900ml		33
Sunflower seeds	120g	A bit under a cup	26

Hemp protein powder (60%)	50g	A bit under half a cup	20
Hemp seeds (hulled)	28g	3 Tablespoons	9
Pea protein powder	50g	A bit under half a cup	18

commercial supplements, including Advital™ (Flavour Creations), Enrich Plus™, Ensure™ (Abbott Nutrition) and Sustagen™ (Nestle Health Sciences)—all available in Australia in 2020—contain leucine in similar levels milk-based powders. Check with manufacturer for more detail (whey protein isolate based powders have higher levels).

Supplement drinks or not?

It is always best to get protein from meals so you also get the benefit of the nutrients in the accompanying foods. However, sometimes you might need to add more than you can easily eat in a meal. This can happen if you are actively working at re-building muscle with an exercise program, trying to recover from an illness or accident, have some major surgery coming up or have recently lost weight you are trying to regain.

High protein drinks (recipes later in this section) or commercial protein supplements can be useful to fill in the gap. The array of supplements in the supermarket aisles can be bewildering, but those based on the dairy product whey (whey protein isolate or whey protein concentrate) are considered to do the best job. If you are vegan or vegetarian you may prefer formulas based on soy or pea protein isolate, or newer options coming onto the market, including hemp protein. You are not going to achieve the body of a Mr, Ms or Mrs Universe, but supplements might just give you the boost your muscles need at times when you are not able to get a good serve of protein at each meal. They can be especially useful as a between meal option so you get the benefits of real food at mealtimes, with the extra boost between.

I don't eat meat—will I get enough protein?

If you have gradually cut down on animal protein foods but are not necessarily committed to vegetarian eating, it is worth reconsidering that choice as you move into older age. As you've heard already, it's generally much easier to get the protein needed from animal foods because their protein concentration means you don't need such large serves as you do from most plant-based protein foods. Animal foods also offer bonus easy-to-access iron, zinc, selenium and vitamin B12.

If you have cut out meat but still eat dairy foods and eggs then you may need to take iron and other supplements if you are not getting enough, but you shouldn't have problems getting the protein you need.

There is no reason at all why you can't get the protein you need as a vegetarian, you just need to be extra vigilant. Closely monitor the protein you eat, as well as making sure you get the other nutrients you need. Nuts, pulses (lentils and beans), seeds, grains and soy products such as tofu are all good options— refer to figure 18 here. Real food is always the best option, but if you need, there are high protein supplements based on soy, rice or other plant proteins like pea protein available to bolster your intake.

A BIT ABOUT ANTIOXIDANTS AS A GROUP

You already know how important antioxidants are, and they gain elevated status the older you get as the tiny bits of oxidative damage accumulate over the years in every cell and organ, including your brain.

Some antioxidants are also vitamins or essential minerals (vitamins A, C and E, selenium and zinc), phytochemicals (substances in plants) but, in a delightfully convenient twist of nature, different ones also happen to provide the colours in different foods. As a basic guide, you really don't need to know much about nutrition to make sure you get plenty of antioxidants: you just need to eat a variety of colours. Ideally, eat at least five or six different coloured foods, or shades of colour, at each meal—more if you can manage it.

Many intensely coloured foods are well known sources of antioxidants: think berries, cherries, red apples, egg yolk, dark green vegetables, green herbs, black olives, multi-coloured lettuce, black and green tea, turmeric and other spices and the wide array of coloured fruits and vegetables, not to mention dark chocolate and red wine! Even pale foods like green and gold apples (both the flesh and the skin), nuts, fish and mushrooms are good sources. You don't need much of each different food you just need to have variety.

Tea (white, green or the more familiar black) is also a great source of a number of antioxidants but it's best drunk between meals, as drinking tea with your meal can reduce your absorption of some other important nutrients, especially iron. Herbal teas and infusions generally contain fewer antioxidant substances and don't cause problems with iron absorption.

Recent research has found that two antioxidant substances,

lutein and zeaxanthin (and their associated xanthans), are especially important for your eyes in helping avoid damage that can lead to cataracts and macular degeneration. These substances are found in dark green vegetables like kale, broccoli and spinach, and the yellow pigments in many foods including eggs.

It also seems that getting antioxidants from foods has the advantage: they are sociable little fellows, much happier working with the team they already know, and may not work as effectively alone as they do when they are in the food they originally came from. So, eating as many different coloured foods as possible is likely to be far more useful than taking individual supplements or consuming huge plates of one vegetable or berry, and it's easy to remember—such an advantage when every one of us worries our memories aren't what they once were!

If the variety of foods you eat dwindles your antioxidant intake also falls. Then it may be tempting to look towards the almost endless variety of commercial antioxidant supplements, drinks and tablets on the market. Advertising claims can be seductive, convincing you that the latest berry or strange-looking fruit from the high Himalayas or darkest Peru has the secret antioxidant to override all others. But the science is clear: none work alone—a combination of many different antioxidants gives the best protection.

VITAMIN A

There are two main forms of vitamin A in foods: retinol found in animal foods and beta-carotene found in yellow and orange fruits and vegetables. It is one of the antioxidant vitamins with an important part to play in cell protection as well in maintaining cognitive function.

Good sources:

> Butter, fortified margarines, organ meats, egg yolks

> Fish liver and fish liver oil (cod liver oil often forced down the throats of children decades ago)

> Yellow and orange fruits and vegetables.

Body:

> Needed to resist infection, keeping skin healthy

> Plays a role in wound healing and cancer prevention

> Essential for good eyesight, especially in low light or at night.

Brain:

> Cell protection

> Deficiency can impact the senses of hearing, taste and smell.

This is not a vitamin most people have to worry about getting enough of, as it's stored in the liver so supply can be maintained through most of life on varying intakes.

As you age changes in the way vitamin A is handled in the body can alter how much is available, particularly to brain cells, and those with long-term issues in the gut, which can impact absorption of fat (such as pancreatic insufficiency, cystic fibrosis and coeliac disease) are at some risk.

As you age, a regular intake is always important. This doesn't mean you should work at getting a lot 'extra' beyond what your body needs. If you type vitamin A into any internet search engine you will get an array of advertising by manufacturers of vitamin supplements and cosmetic companies for its 'anti-ageing'/brain boosting/ antioxidant capabilities/skin benefits and more. Think carefully and ask your doctor or dietitian before you take any supplements because excess accumulates in the liver and is toxic. That includes over enthusiastic intake of the liver of oily fish or oil from them (including cod liver oil).

Vitamin A toxicity can cause skin changes, dryness of lips, nasal passages and eyes, peeling of skin, hair loss and nail fragility, irritability, glare sensitivity, vertigo, loss of appetite and abnormal liver function. Research has found that taking (unnecessary) supplements long term increases the risk of hip fracture in older women, which might be worse if their vitamin D levels are low (especially if vitamin A is in the form of retinal, retinol or retinoic acid).

You might be interested to know that vitamin A toxicity is widely thought to have contributed to or finally caused the deaths of Antarctic explorers Douglas Mawson and Xavier Metz who were forced to eat the livers of their Husky dogs, subsequently found to be very high in this vitamin.

Even a multivitamin containing vitamin A beyond recommended levels could, over time, create problems. Any supplement you pick up should indicate on the label how much of the RDA (Recommended Dietary Allowance) each contains. Unless you are taking something specifically prescribed to correct a deficiency, you should avoid taking more than the RDA of any substance. I know many people like to take a multivitamin 'just to be sure' and if you do, I would suggest choosing something providing about 50% of the RDA—the rest should come from food.

It's also important if you take anticoagulant medication (to prevent blood clots—often prescribed after a heart attack or stroke), to be aware that taking vitamin A supplements can increase their effects and cause excessive bleeding. Always check any supplements you take with your doctor—just because you buy something without a prescription doesn't mean it is harmless.

Fortunately, as long as you eat a good variety of foods containing vitamin A, especially plenty of yellow and orange vegetables and fruits, it's unusual to run into either a deficiency or excess.

This is definitely one you need to check with your doctor and/or dietitian.

VITAMIN C

Good sources:

> Citrus fruits

> Capsicum and other peppers

> Cabbage.

Other sources:

> Leafy vegetables – especially dark green.

Body:

> Essential to heal wounds

> Keep teeth, gums and bones healthy

> Important antioxidant—protects vitamin E and folate from degradation

> Helps fight infection and assists in getting iron from food.

Brain:

> Needed to make neurotransmitters

> Low levels are associated with reduced cognitive abilities.

There have been numerous claims made over the years about the benefits of taking high doses of this vitamin in tablet or powder form and most recently suggesting it can protect against dementia. While it certainly is essential in that, it is unlikely to act in the same way when removed from its original food source. It's possible the many other substances that exist with it in those foods also have antioxidant properties and roles to play. It is likely that, when separated, they do not work as they originally did.

VITAMIN E

Good sources:

> Nuts and seeds, and oils made from them

> Wheatgerm

> Egg yolk.

Other sources:

> Avocado

> Leafy vegetables.

Body:

> Maintains health in all body cells

> Plays a central role in immune defence and assists in wound healing

> Plays a central role in protecting all cells from cancer and heart problems.

Brain:

> Promotes efficient blood flow through the brain—nourishing and protecting cells

> Cell protection and immune response

> Low levels are associated with reduced memory and cognitive ability.

Vitamin E is one of the most powerful nutritional antioxidants so has many roles throughout the body and brain. As a result supplement tablets are heavily promoted as being protective and boosting cognition but sadly, the benefits don't stack up as many would hope. Again, it may be a case of natural food being the best source.

Deficiency is not very common, although it can happen in some illnesses, especially where there is chronic diarrhoea or malabsorption because it is a vitamin that is absorbed from foods along with fat and that is poorly absorbed when these occur.

If your appetite is down, your food intake is low or you experience long-term loose bowels/diarrhoea (even if intermittent), this is one to ask your doctor about.

VITAMIN D

Good sources:

> The most important source is that made under your skin when it's exposed to sunlight

> Pink fleshed fish (such as salmon and ocean trout)

> Oily fish (mackerel, sardines), cod liver and cod liver oil (take care with these last two—you've already read about them under vitamin A).

Other sources:

> Egg yolk

> Natural butter (levels are lower in most 'soft' versions), fortified margarine

> Mushrooms that have had time in the sun (field grown) or have been irradiated with UV light (available in some stores and labelled as such). Fun fact about mushrooms: you can add vitamin D to any mushrooms, even those purchased in a supermarket, by putting them in the sun, smooth side up, for just five or ten minutes then store as usual. They hold the vitamin D until you eat them—so clever!

Body:

> Essential for bone mineralisation (laying down minerals including calcium)

> Important for an effective immune response to infection

> Deficiency causes weakness and pain in large muscles, affecting activity levels

> Helps maintain healthy blood pressure

> Deficiency contributes to heart disease, certain cancers (colorectal, breast and prostate), diabetes.

Brain:

> Protection of neurons—including assisting with clearance of beta amyloid from the brain

> Cardiovascular benefits—including reducing stiffening and atherosclerotic plaque build up in blood vessels

> Blood pressure benefits—help protect small brain blood vessels

> Involved in plasticity.

Deficiency of vitamin D is a problem affecting up to one third of people in Australia and is more likely in older age. In hostels and aged care facilities, the figure jumps to over half of residents!

While we don't yet know exactly how it works in the brain, its role in there is undeniable because there are specific receptors within the brain for vitamin D and its metabolites. We know it is involved in plasticity, in the survival of neurones and in transmission of information, and it is thought to play a role in depression and anxiety—both of which impact on cognitive abilities in the short or long term.

Unlike most vitamins, you only get small amounts of vitamin D from foods. Most of what you need is produced through your skin when you are in the sun and that production can be less efficient as you age. Now that we don't get the same sun exposure our forebears did, we risk not getting enough vitamin D.

If you tend to be involved in mostly indoor activities, work indoors, find it difficult to get outside, or choose to avoid the sun for other reasons such as skin cancer concerns, then you are very likely not getting enough vitamin D. If you are out and about every day, gardening, fishing, walking or doing other similar outdoor activities and exposing at least your arms and some of your legs and face without sunscreen for about half an hour most days, then you might be able to get what you need, but for anyone else, and during winter especially, choosing foods with vitamin D and adding supplements to make up any shortfall is the way to go.

If you're not sure, ask your doctor to arrange a blood test to have your vitamin D status assessed. If your levels are just a bit low, or if they are fine but you're not getting any sun, a low dose supplement each day is probably needed. If you are found to be deficient you may need quite a lot more; and it can take a few months to get levels back up.

If you have bone density concerns and don't get a good calcium intake, then a supplement combining calcium and vitamin D may be suggested by your doctor or dietitian.

As far as excess intake goes, that's not likely from most foods, but do take care if you are a fan of cod liver oil or the liver of oily fish (such as canned cod liver). These are high in vitamin D, but also in vitamin A and the latter can be a problem as you have read. People sometimes eat such foods for their very high omega-3 content but they need to be considered as if they were a medication due to the chance they can cause vitamin A toxicity.

VITAMIN B1 (THIAMINE)

Good sources:

> Many cereal foods are fortified with thiamin, including breakfast cereals, commercial breads, malted drinks like AktaviteTM, MiloTM, OvaltineTM

> Yeast extract spreads including VegemiteTM, MarmiteTM

> Nuts—especially cashews, peanuts, brazil nuts

> Liver, kidney, lean pork meat.

Body:

> Supports a healthy appetite

> Helps detoxify alcohol—deficiency is most common in excessive alcohol consumption.

Brain:

> Important in communication between neurons.

Thiamine plays a vital role in neurotransmission, so is indispensable in the brain. As we have no way of storing this vitamin it must be eaten daily, but deficiency is rare in most western countries because it's found in so many foods. However, deficiency is possible if food intake is low for a while and it can develop in people who drink excessive amounts of alcohol because it is also used in the detoxification of alcohol in the body.

VITAMIN B3 (NIACIN)

Good sources:

> Similar to B1 (fortified breakfast cereals, nuts, chicken meat, liver, wholegrains).

Body:

> Helps fuel all cells—breakdown of nutrients, energy release, oxygen use.

Brain:

> Helps make neurotransmitters.

Niacin often works in combination with the other B group vitamins (thiamine B1 and riboflavin B2) and can be made in the body from the amino acid tryptophan; its role in neurotransmitter production makes it especially important for the brain.

There have been many claims that niacin is a wonder nutrient for the brain and, more traditionally, for heart function. Unfortunately, many of these claims are inflated and it's important to avoid taking too much because excess can cause problems also. Vitamin B3 is certainly essential to brain function; and some people have used it to assist in managing heart disease, but only under strict medical supervision to avoid causing other problems.

Although it's important to get enough B3, a deficiency is rare unless you've been eating poorly for quite some time, and then it will be only one of many nutrients lacking.

VITAMIN B6 (PYRIDOXINE)

Good sources:

> Lean meats, liver, poultry, oily fish

> Pulses including lentils, kidney beans, lima beans

> Nuts, sunflower seeds

> Eggplant (aubergine), silverbeet, bok choy.

Body:

> Helps the body use proteins and carbohydrate fuel

> Assists in formation of red blood cells.

Brain:

> Assists in keeping homocysteine (see figure 20 below) levels in a helpful range (with folate and B12).

Figure 20: A note on homocysteine

If you read a bit on health you may have heard mention of homocysteine and how it's bad for your heart and might cause stroke and Alzheimer's disease, which is certainly true if the levels in your blood are too high.

Homocysteine in just the right amount has an important role to play too. It comes from the proteins we eat and, with the help of the vitamins folate, B6 and B12, is used to make two substances that are very good for you, one of which is a powerful antioxidant called glutathione.

It's only a problem when homocysteine doesn't get converted into glutathione, which happens if your levels of these B vitamins are too low, so it builds up in your blood. Keeping homocysteine levels just right depends on making sure you don't become deficient, but unfortunately taking extra vitamins beyond that doesn't add extra benefit. You might hear some big claims made that various supplements reduce homocysteine levels; always check with your doctor before taking these vitamins in tablet form. Taking them when you are not deficient can cause you harm.

There are also supplements of glutathione itself with claims that it will help but, sadly, the reality is that these don't get absorbed well enough to be of much use, despite their considerable cost, so will probably give you little or no benefit.

B6 is important in assisting brain activity and a deficiency may be linked to depression, but it also plays an integral part in regulating levels of homocysteine and has recently been touted as helping to avoid Alzheimer's disease partly because of this, but take care because high doses can damage nerve endings.

Like all vitamins you need just the right amount, excess can be as damaging as not enough.

Fortunately, deficiency is not common as it's in a lot of foods. Eating poorly over a long period puts you at most risk.

FOLATE (FOLIC ACID)

Note that folate is the natural form of this vitamin, found naturally in a variety of foods, while folic acid is the synthetic form used in supplements and added to foods like bread and breakfast cereals. Folic acid, despite not being the most 'natural form', is considered to be more easily absorbed than folate.

Good sources:

> Darker green vegetables and leafy greens (kale, spinach, Asian vegetables, broccoli)

> Liver, kidney

> Fortified breakfast cereals, breads and juices with added folate.

Other sources:

> Nuts, chickpeas, and yeast

> Vegetable extracts such as Vegemite and Marmite.

Body:

> Has a vital role in all dividing cells (building and maintenance)

> Formation of red blood cells

> May help prevent age-related hearing loss and macular degeneration

> Assists in prevention of colon/bowel cancer.

Brain:

> Deficiency is well known to have cognitive impacts across all stages of life

> Low body levels significantly increase chance of developing Alzheimer's dementia.

Low folate status can cause blood levels of homocysteine to rise, but when allowed to accumulate in the bloodstream, it is associated with heart disease and Alzheimer's dementia.

Luckily folate (as folic acid) is found in a lot of foods, and if you eat well you'll usually be okay but problems can crop up because some common medications interfere with the way folate is used (see figure 21 below). If you take any of these medications for more than a week you should have your folate status checked regularly by your doctor, as you may need supplements or other interventions if your levels are too low.

Figure 21: Medications that may affect folate status (brand names in *italics*)

Metformin for diabetes	including *Diabex, Diaformin, Formet, Glucobet, Glucophage, Glucophage XR, Metex*
Sulphasalazine used in cases of Irritable Bowel Syndrome, Crohn's disease and Ulcerative Colitis	including *Salazopyrin, Salazopyrin SR, Pyralin EN*
Phenytoin anticonvulsant/anti epileptic	*Dilantin*

Methotrexate used in cancer therapy and rheumatoid arthritis	*Methoblastin*
Triamterene, a diuretic	including *Hydrene 25/50*
Barbiturates (sedatives not often	other names are amylobarbitone and amobarbital used nowadays)
Some blood lipid lowering fibrates	including Fenofibrate (*Lipidil*)
NSAIDS (Non-steroidal anti-inflammatory) medications for mild or moderate pain, fever and inflammation relief	available without prescription—including ibuprofen (*Nurofen, Advil* and generics) naproxen (*Naprosyn*), and aspirin
	others available only on prescription include diclofenac (*Voltaren*), celecoxib (*Celebrex*), meloxicam (*Mobic*), piroxicam (*Feldene*), indomethacin (*Indocid*), mefanamic acid (*Ponstan*), ketoprofen (*Orudis*)

The common NSAID (non steroidal anti inflammatory drug) pain relievers including ibuprophen and aspirin and others mentioned in **figure 21**, are worth a special mention. Since they can be bought at a supermarket or chemist without a prescription, many people believe them to be completely safe and may take them often enough to affect folate levels. If you do take them regularly without a script, let your doctor know; you may need to try alternative medications or take folate supplements if there is an issue. Other NSAIDs cause similar problems but are only available on prescription, and your doctor can easily monitor them.

Paracetamol [Panadol and generics] is a different type of pain relief medication and does not cause the same issues.

Very low dose aspirin such as Cartia 100 and Cardiprin 100 brands are often prescribed to help reduce 'stickiness' in the blood, most often after a heart attack or stroke to avoid a recurrence, but also as a prevention. These low dose tablets may not cause the problems higher doses of most NSAIDs do, but your folate status should be monitored regularly if you take them routinely. Take care if you have chosen to take low dose aspirin without a prescription and are in your 70s or beyond because they might increase your chance of experiencing ulcers or bleeding in your stomach or upper gastrointestinal tract– as with all medications, keep discussing what's still needed as you age with your doctor.

A severe folate deficiency can cause diarrhoea, loss of appetite, weight loss, weakness, sore tongue, headaches, heart palpitations, irritability and forgetfulness.

Before you think of taking folate as a tablet, a word of caution: first get a test to check if you are deficient, because getting too much folate on its own can worsen kidney problems or hide the signs of a damaging vitamin B12 deficiency.

Be extra careful if you have reduced kidney function, taking high doses of folate alone or in very high doses with other B vitamins in tablet form can worsen any kidney damage. While most lower-dose combined B vitamin supplements contain both folate and B12 in amounts that won't cause you harm, you must always discuss taking any vitamin or mineral supplement tablet with your doctor to avoid extra problems.

VITAMIN B12

Good sources:

> Animal foods of all types: meat, poultry, dairy foods, eggs, seafood.

Other sources (smaller amounts):

> Fortified soy milk

> Mushrooms

> Fermented foods containing live yeasts and bacteria.

Body:

> Formation of red blood cells

> Maintaining health of nerves throughout the body

> Energy metabolism.

Brain:

> Needed for correct functioning of neurons

> Energy supply to all brain cells.

B12 and folate together help maintain homocysteine at a safe level.

Vitamin B12 deficiency is worryingly common in older age, and can be mistaken for dementia because symptoms include confusion, difficulty in concentrating, memory loss, irritability and depression. Other signs of deficiency include anaemia, fatigue, shortness of breath, tingling and numbness in the limbs, loss of balance, loss of bladder and bowel control and reduced appetite.

There are some likely reasons why B12 deficiency is so common:

1. Avoiding dementia diagnosis/delaying treatment: it's not surprising that someone might want to avoid being diagnosed with dementia if they find themselves facing becoming confused or forgetting things. However, if the problem is B12 deficiency, that's treatable and they can get better! If, on the other hand, treatment is delayed, permanent damage to the brain and nervous system can result and that is an avoidable tragedy.

2. Malabsorption issues: B12 needs just the right amount of acid from your stomach to allow it to be absorbed from the gut but, as you get older age-related changes in your stomach and intestines can reduce acid levels so, even if you are eating foods containing enough B12, it doesn't make it to your blood system. If you suffer recurrent gastrointestinal upset or diarrhoea, as you may in irritable bowel syndrome, as a side effect of antibiotics or due to other illness, you can miss out on your B12.

3. Medication issues: commonly prescribed PPI (Proton Pump Inhibitor—see **figure 22**) medications for reflux are designed to reduce acid production in your stomach. That can also impact B12 absorption and deficiency can happen in time. Pharmacists generally advise most people taking these not to stay on them long term, but many people do. Another that can impact B12 is the diabetes medication Metformin. If you have been taking a PPI or Metformin (especially for more than a few years), or are concerned, ask your doctor to test your B12 levels. Regular testing identifies

if there is a problem, which can then be treated.

4. Reducing intake of animal foods: last but certainly not least, if you gradually cut down on eating meat and other animal foods as you get older, you might set yourself up for a B12 deficiency.

As with folate, most people easily get enough B12 in their diet, but these above issues can mess with that. If any apply to you, or if you take medications listed in **figure 22,** you must have your B12 levels checked regularly so any deficiency can be quickly corrected. Fortunately that just means a simple blood test and, should that identify a deficiency, it is completely reversible if treated promptly.

Figure 22: Anti reflux medications and B12:

List of common anti-reflux medications, which may affect B12 levels when used over a number of years:

The PPIs (proton pump inhibitors):

Esomeprazole (Nexium)   Lansoprazole (Zoton)

Omeprazole (Losec, Prohibitor)

Pantoprazole (Somac)

Rabprazole (Pariet)

The H2 blockers are less likely to cause problems but also reduce stomach acid so having B12 status checked is prudent in late age:

Ranitidine (Zantac, Rani,Ranitidine)

Cimetidine (Tagamet)

Nizatidine (Tazac)

Famotidine (Amfamox, Pepcidine)

VITAMIN K

Vitamin K is important to mention because of its interaction with the blood-thinning medication Warfarin (brand names include Coumadin and Marevan in Australia) many older people take.

Good sources:

> Green vegetables

> Also made by gut bacteria.

Other sources (smaller amounts):

> Meat and dairy foods

> Berries.

Body:

> Clots blood to stop bleeding when your skin is damaged

> Helps prevent bone fracture and reduces bone loss in postmenopausal women

> Helps avoid 'hardening' of blood vessels.

Vitamin K has an essential role in stopping massive loss of blood after relatively minor injury, but some medical conditions can cause blood to clot inside your blood vessels when it shouldn't, putting you at risk of stroke or heart attack. To avoid this, or if you have already suffered such an event, you may be prescribed warfarin.

Warfarin works by acting against vitamin K in the body. The amount of warfarin you take is balanced against your vitamin K intake to get your rate of blood clotting just right for your condition (the degree of clotting is assessed by the INR blood test, done regularly once you are on this medication).

Many people who take warfarin believe they must stop eating foods with vitamin K to get their INR right, but that is wrong— it is a balance that's needed. The foods that contain vitamin K also supply a lot of other essential nutrients (like folate, vitamin C and many different antioxidants), so cutting them out is just not a good idea. What you need to do is plan to eat about the same amount of food containing vitamin K each day, and then your dose of warfarin gets balanced against that.

Balancing food sources of vitamin K

Choose a selection from this list each day (the quantities provide about the same amount of vitamin K):

Asian greens (all varieties): ⬚ cup cooked

Asparagus: 8 medium spears

Beetroot leaves (NOT the beetroot itself): ⬚ cup

Broccoli: 1/2 cup cooked

Cabbage (darker green/red varieties): 1 cup

Endive: 1 cup

Fresh, green herbs (basil, coriander, rocket, parsley): approx. 1/2 cup in total should be counted, but amounts less than that, included as part of a recipe for more than just one person, or used as garnish, pose no problem

Kale: 1/2 cup cooked

Lettuce ('fancy', darker types): 1 cup

Spinach/silverbeet: 1/2 cup cooked

Mix these foods up as you wish, but make sure you get approximately the same amount of vitamin K- containing food each day. To maintain variety, perhaps have a mix of broccoli and kale one day, spinach another, mix coleslaw with four spears of asparagus another, and a stir-fry with Asian greens on another day.

It shouldn't really affect your INR at all if you are only having a sprinkle or a teaspoon of herbs (or even if you use half a cup in a dish for a few people), one or two asparagus spears, a few bits of broccoli in a stir fry or a scattering of dark green or red lettuce in a salad mix.

There are also herbal preparations and supplements, which although they don't contain vitamin K, can affect your INR in other ways. If you are considering taking any of these, discuss it first with your doctor or dietitian.

Chamomile (in large amounts, not an occasional cup of tea)

Cranberry juice (more than one glass a day)

Omega-3 supplements (such as fish oil)

Garlic capsules (this means high dose garlic in a capsule, not what you have in meals unless you eat a number of whole cloves at once)

Gingko biloba, ginseng, fenugreek tablets

Green tea in large amounts

Iron, magnesium or zinc supplements (usually okay if taken two hours before or after warfarin)

Glucosamine, chondroitin (usually taken for joint pain)

Vitamin E in large doses

CALCIUM

Good Sources:

> Dairy foods—milk, yoghurt, cheese but not cream or butter

> Soy and other milks with added calcium

> Fish with edible bones (such as canned salmon or sardines).

Other sources (smaller amounts):

> Sesame seeds and some nuts (almonds, brazil nuts, hazelnuts)

> Dried figs

> Broccoli.

Body:

> Builds and maintains strong bones

> Involved in muscle activity

> Vital role in heart contraction.

You have read a bit about calcium in Bodyworks, looking at bone health and it is important to reiterate that getting calcium from food also requires vitamin D to absorb and use it properly. It's also vital to consider and discuss your individual situation with your doctor before deciding to take a high dose of calcium because medical research has found that high dose calcium alone can cause heart problems.

You may lose calcium if you eat too much salt, because that can cause the kidneys to get rid of calcium unnecessarily. Ideally, some dairy food at each meal, plus at least one extra calcium food per day should be adequate for most people and provide the balance to avoid such losses.

If you do take calcium supplements, don't take huge amounts and choose one that also includes vitamin D to help absorption.

What's the latest about salt in foods?

Processing food by adding salt (everyday salt contains sodium and that's what is significant) in the past when refrigeration was inadequate or less widely available was an extremely important way of keeping food for as long as possible. We got used to that flavour and anyone who grew up eating salted meat and other foods preserved with salt will attest to its appeal. That doesn't mean those are bad foods it just means that more and more we need to balance the ones that have salt, and to some extent sugars, added for their preservation (or more so nowadays to give them a taste that appeals to our salt flavour sensors) with fresh fruits, vegetables, nuts, seeds, meat and dairy foods that are naturally low in salt.

Food processing often adds salt to accommodate the taste requirements of consumers, so eating an excessive amount of foods that have undergone processing from their original form can add to the salt load in the body. Is that a problem?

For many years advice has consistently advocated a low-salt diet for a range of health benefits, but a recent wide-ranging review of the evidence by the Institute of Medicine in the US (an independent collaboration of research experts) found that both very high and low levels were problematic. What was more significant than sodium (in regular salt) was the amount of potassium. It seems as long as your potassium intake is good, it is less important how much sodium you get.

The same goes for those experiencing Meniere's disease: a distressing problem where the fluid balance in the inner ear is disrupted causing vertigo (dizziness) and other challenging symptoms. A restricted salt diet can be helpful for many people with this disease, but again getting the potassium needed is also important. (There are links to more information on Meniere's in the Further Reading section at the end of the book)

As potassium is found in many foods—especially fruits and vegetables—there are many benefits to eating extra potassium because of the antioxidants they also contain. (see the list below)

The thing about enjoying the salt taste is that the more salt you eat, the more you need in order to enjoy foods in the same way. If you cut down, you need to do it gradually so you get used to the change and your enjoyment continues.

Remember that your sense of taste declines with age so you might actually need more salt or other flavours in foods to be able to appreciate them as you always have done. If food tastes like nothing and that means you find it a challenge to eat, then adding salt to foods might be what's needed to ward off malnutrition. It's always a balance and it's always a matter for each individual to consider quality of life and weigh up what's really important.

For anyone already living with dementia it may be that adding extra salt to encourage intake and enjoyment and avoid the far more dangerous problems that weight loss can cause might just be the answer—add potassium-containing foods where possible to give an extra benefit.

Foods high in potassium: most yellow or orange fruits (particularly bananas) and vegetables, tomatoes, legumes, lentils and dried beans of all types, broccoli, kale, Brussels sprouts, dried fruits, milk and dairy foods, nuts and seeds and chocolate.

IODINE

Good sources:

> High levels in seaweed and anything that contains seaweed (nori) including sushi

> Most seafood, especially shellfish,

> Foods prepared with iodised salt (salt that has had iodine added).

Body:

> Vital for thyroid function and regulation of body processes.

Brain:

> Essential for development and correct functioning of neurons, glia and neuronal connections throughout life (deficiency during pregnancy causes mental retardation in children).

The amount of iodine that foods contain depends on how much is in the soil, and in Australia and many other countries unfortunately those levels are low. Most iodine people get now comes from the oceans.

Years ago, iodine was commonly added to table salt to boost the amount people ate, but now people often avoid salt or eat 'gourmet' salt (sea salt crystals, pink salt), which don't contain iodine. We also used to get a lot from milk and dairy foods as a by-product of the use of iodine-based cleaning products in dairies; but those products are rarely used now, so dairy foods don't supply the iodine they once did. Some older books and lists of iodine-containing foods suggest dairy foods as a good source but that is no longer the case.

You may also be aware that iodine is used in skin sterilising solutions, applied before a surgical procedure, and in products you can purchase to use at home to treat wounds and in throat gargles. These are not intended for consumption. Such products contain povidone-iodine and while you can potentially absorb small amounts from wounds or swallow some if you are using it as a gargle to treat a sore throat, those are usually not significant because use is short term. Long-term use in open wounds or similar can potentially cause overdose however, so ask the advice of a healthcare professional in such cases.

Overdose is not common from food but do take care if you have a huge passion for sushi or Japanese seaweed salad. In cultures that traditionally eat these foods, seaweed-containing foods are only part of meals, often as small side dishes, so intake is not usually excessive. If you suddenly decide you must have a few sushi rolls or seaweed salad every day, you may get more than is helpful.

If you don't eat seafood or consume seaweed products regularly, then make sure you use iodised salt or one of the 'gourmet' varieties that combine ground seaweed with sea salt. If none of these apply, get your doctor to check your blood levels—a supplement may be required.

A special note for people with thyroid conditions:

A number of conditions that are not diet related can impact thyroid function. In hypothyroidism (an under active thyroid) production of thyroid hormones is too low; in hyperthyroidism (over active) it is too high. Either can be damaging and require medical treatment to supply the right amount of these hormones that are essential to body and brain function.

Hashimoto's disease usually causes hypothyroidism (but can sometimes swing into hyperthyroidism), while Graves disease is associated with hyperthyroidism. Sometimes cancer in the thyroid requires its surgical removal or radiation treatment that impacts its capacity to produce these hormones also.

In none of these medical conditions is diet the cause of the problem, but what you eat can impact how well the medical treatment for your condition works. That particularly applies to eating large amounts of soy foods or taking iron supplements close to when you have certain thyroid medications. There is a link to more on this in the Further Reading and Resources section, but ask your doctor and you can always seek the advice of a dietitian to assist.

IRON

Good sources:

> Red meats (liver and kidney are highest)

> Pork, poultry and seafood.

Other sources (smaller amounts):

> Dark green leafy vegetables,

> Soy foods, lentils, eggs, seeds

> Fortified breakfast cereals.

Body:

> Required to make haemoglobin in red blood cells for oxygen supply to all cells.

Brain:

> Required to make neurotransmitters

> Oxygen supply to all brain cells

> Assists in protections of neurons.

Most people know that you become anaemic if your iron levels fall too low, but what you may not know is that a mild iron deficiency, which isn't even obvious without a blood test, can contribute to reduced cognition. Since the brain does so much its oxygen needs are high, so even a minor shortfall means it can't function properly. If that shortfall continues, permanent damage happens.

There are three things that can set you up for iron deficiency. The first are medical conditions that cause you to lose blood (from chronic ulcers in your stomach or upper intestine, anything which causes blood loss from the bowel—including bowel cancer—bleeding gums, or frequent cuts, bruises and grazes). Second is any medical issue or medication that reduces your ability to absorb iron from food. And last, but certainly not least because it's so very common, is gradually cutting down on eating high iron foods like red meat.

Iron, like vitamin B12, needs stomach acid for efficient absorption, and you have read how that declines with age and medications. Surprisingly, some food and drinks make it more difficult to get iron from your meals. Tea is one, so, as you get older if you tend to have low iron levels it's very important to avoid drinking tea at the same time as your meals. Leave at least an hour between eating a meal and having your cup of tea (that doesn't apply to green tea, herbal tea, infusions or coffee).

It can take many months or years for your iron levels to get low enough to cause even a mild deficiency, but if any of the above are familiar to you, make sure you have regular blood tests.

Prevention is, as always, prudent. From now on make sure you get iron-containing foods a few days a week: liver (lambs fry), kidney, red meats, poultry and fish are the best sources. Vegetarians should be especially vigilant.

Iron has been found to accumulate in the brain and that may contribute to cognitive issues but eating iron-containing food is probably not the issue as you read in Brainworks.

ZINC

Good sources:

> Oysters are far higher than any other food

> Red meats and wild meats, a bit less in pork, chicken and fish.

Other sources:

> Fortified breakfast cereals (zinc added during manufacture)

> Nuts, seeds, peas.

Body:

> Important in infection resistance, wound healing and in regulating many body processes

> Deficiency impacts appetite and reduces sense of taste and smell.

Brain:

> Vital in creating and maintaining brain cells and in neurotransmission

Some medications can bind zinc in the gut, making it unavailable for absorption by the body and potentially causing deficiency in the long term, especially if food intake should reduce with age. One group are the thiazide diuretics (check with your doctor or pharmacist) for blood pressure: these contain hydrochlorothiazide, indapamide or related substances with brand names in Australia including Atacand plus, Monoplus, Moduretic, Avapro and Natrilix.

Zinc is second only to iron in content in the brain and inadequate intake is linked to reduced memory, learning ability and impaired cognition. But get too much and—a bit like iron—it may play a part in the development of dementia by contributing to accumulation of βamyloid, so balance is absolutely essential.

Fortunately getting too much from food is unlikely unless you eat nothing but oysters all the time!

However, taking zinc in tablets, alone or combined with other vitamins/minerals increases the likelihood. You might take these believing you need help with wound healing, fighting infections, improving your sense of taste or your appetite; or use them with other nutrients like vitamin C, vitamin E and beta-carotene to help avoid macular degeneration. And yes, zinc is important for all those things, but it's only needed in small amounts, and unless you are actually deficient, taking more than is needed could cause problems instead of preventing or curing them. More is not better with nutrient minerals, no matter what the marketing people say.

Even multivitamin/mineral tablets, if taken when you don't really need them, can contribute, so always check with your doctor. You really only need to take higher dose tablets when you know you are deficient, to get your levels up where they should be.

Like iron, your body accesses and regulates zinc best when you get it from animal foods so vegetarians need to be careful.

Plant sources of zinc often contain a type of fibre that holds on to the zinc so it is passed out in your faeces instead of being absorbed into the blood.

MAGNESIUM

Good sources:

> Soy beans and soy foods

> Nuts and nut butters

> Seeds, rice and wheat bran

> Whole grains and foods made with them

> Molasses, treacle and dark sugars (dark brown sugar and similar)

> Sweetcorn, maize and products made from them.

Other sources (smaller amounts):

> Dark green vegetables

> Sundried tomatoes

> Milk powder

> Fish

Body:

> Coordination of muscle contraction and production of healthy bone

> Assists nerve transmission

> Helps maintain heart rhythm

> Involved in releasing energy from food, building protein for muscle tissue

> Assists in blood glucose control.

Brain:

> Assists neurotransmitter release from neurons

> Vital in mitochondrial function (energy supply)

> Involved in removal of βamyloid from the brain.

Magnesium is a remarkable nutrient, active in a huge number of body processes. Even without deficiency, an inadequate intake may contribute to chronic inflammation and oxidative stress in body and brain.

In the brain its role in the release of neurotransmitters and the work of mitochondria, which are the power supply systems in each cell, mean any issues with its availability can quickly affect your brain's capacity. That poses two particular problems for older people.

The first is to do with our eating habits and food processing. Magnesium is concentrated in the outer layers of grains and in minimally refined foods, so our modern diet tends to provide less than it once did. It also needs to be in the soil to get into vegetables, so unless vegetables are grown in good soil they can be low in magnesium. Stick with whole grain foods for their fibre and add some soy products, nuts and seeds, and you will get magnesium too.

The second problem has to do with how well it is retained in the body. Unfortunately, even if it's in food, magnesium gets more difficult to absorb with age because of changes in the gut and an increased tendency of the kidneys to pass it out in the urine. Medications that also have an impact on this mineral include the 'loop diuretics' (common brand names in Australia are Frusemide, Lasix and Urex) and some antibiotics.

It is thought that vitamin D helps in its absorption, so if that is low too getting enough magnesium can have added challenges.

This is another mineral to take care with if you are considering a supplement, because higher doses cause diarrhoea (milk of magnesia is an old-fashioned cure-all for indigestion and constipation—it contains magnesium hydroxide—epsom salt is magnesium sulfate and works the same way). Lower dose tablets are usually fine, but always check with your doctor first as it can interact with some medications.

SELENIUM

Good sources:

> Nuts (especially brazil nuts)

> Fish, seafood, liver, kidney, red meat, chicken, eggs

> Mushrooms and grains (the level of selenium in foods usually depends on how much is in the soil from which they are sourced and soils in Australia are low).

Body:

> Powerful antioxidant properties

> Bolsters the effects of some other antioxidant substances including vitamin C

> Immune system regulator

> Assists thyroid function.

Brain:

> Protection of all brain cells.

Selenium has made health news in recent years with the discovery that people who have better selenium status have better brain health and that there is a possibility that it helps fight some cancers, especially prostate cancer. The understandable desire to avoid prostate cancer may lead some people to take large amounts of selenium but getting too much is just as much a problem as too little because it's toxic in high doses.

If you are concerned that you might not be getting enough, always get your doctor to check your selenium status; but getting it from food presents few problems.

OMEGA-3 FATS (FATTY ACIDS)

Fat is not always the bad guy. It's a normal component of many natural foods, including meats, dairy foods, nuts, seeds, oils, grains and some vegetables; and it carries many of the flavour components of foods. It gives foods a creamy mouth feel and, importantly, is great at keeping appetite up to scratch at a time in life when eating may lose its interest.

Omega-3 fats are a type of polyunsaturated fat that we cannot make ourselves so must get from the food we eat. There are three of note: DHA (docosahexanoic acid), EPA (eicosapentaenioc acid) and ALA (alpha-linolenic acid).

Good sources:

> DHA and EPA: Oily fish (salmon, tuna, mackerel, sardines), fish liver and its oil

> Smaller amounts in grass fed meats, wild meats (kangaroo or rabbit), egg yolks

> ALA: flax seeds, chia, walnuts and pecans, silverbeet, broccoli and spinach.

Body:

> Reduces the effects of atherosclerosis in blood vessels and help them stay flexible

> Balances the cardio-protective roles of other fats.

Brain:

> Blood vessel benefits, also important for the brain

> DHA found in high concentrations in brain—involved in transmission of nerve signals

> EPA, ALA involved in energy supply to brain cells.

Many generations ago when mostly wild or free ranging animals were eaten, these unsaturated fats were much more common in our diets. You can still get them from oily fish, wild or game meats, meat and milk from animals that graze pastures freely rather than eat grain in paddocks, as well as from some nuts and seeds and their oils. A large amount of the food we eat contains little or none, or has other oil and food components that reduce how much we get.

Due to this, omega-3 supplements (including fish oil, krill oil, flaxseed oil) are extraordinarily popular. Most on the market in 2020 are extracted from high omega-3 plant seeds and marine animals such as small ocean fish and krill (the very small sea creatures eaten by whales).

There has been quite a bit of research on omega-3 and that continues. Many scientists suggest taking high doses of omega-3, but common sense is important. It's tempting to think that if omega-3 fatty acids are important to the brain, and that our modern diets don't readily supply them, then taking as much as possible in supplement form will always be good. But, like everything, a balance is prudent. One reason is that omega-3s are also contributors to oxidation reactions in cells, which means oxidative waste will be produced in the process.

Unless antioxidant intake is high enough to balance very high intakes, the net result could be harmful, not helpful.

Also, should you choose to supplement what you get from food by taking omega-3 as fish or krill oil, keep in mind that it can take many, many kilograms of small fish or krill from the ocean to make just one kilogram of the oil in those tablets, so be sure you are not taking more than you really need.

ALA has been thought of as a poor cousin to DHA and EPA because experiments in laboratories found it didn't seem to convert well into the DHA the brain needs. This was confusing because despite the claims of manufacturers of fish oil supplements that these are unique for maintaining DHA levels in the brain, vegetarians who don't eat fish and vegans who eat no animal products at all do not have very low levels and do not develop dementia in greater numbers, so there had to be something else involved.

It is now believed that people who get most or all of their omega-3 fats from ALA are very good at making that conversion, while those who regularly eat oily fish or get plenty of DHA/EPA in other ways, don't need to so it doesn't happen as much, if at all.

FOODWORKS

PART 2

Eating Plans to Guide Your Day

*T*he aim of the plans in this chapter is to offer suggestions of the best options for your health and life stage. Choose the plan that suits your stage of life and always vary the foods you eat.

PLAN 1: FOR THOSE WHO ARE MAINLY IN GOOD HEALTH AND HAVEN'T UNINTENTIONALLY LOST WEIGHT

This is a guide to the sorts of foods you should include at each meal to help your muscles and brain, and relies on you doing exercise. If you are not active then you need to find ways to become so. You must work to build and maintain muscle at the same time as eating. You need to balance activity with what you eat to avoid gaining weight, or get additional advice from a dietitian.

The list here has a selection of foods containing protein and other foods from which you can choose your meals. Figure 20 in Foodworks gave you an idea of the quantities of foods needed to get 20g: you can use that to make combinations for more or less as required.

If you have low appetite days or are not feeling 100%, you may need to eat according to Plan 2 or 3, at least for a while. At such times it's fine to have:

> High protein drinks instead of a meal

> Only desserts, as long as they are higher protein desserts

> Only soups, provided they are higher protein soups

> Or even tea and toast for a short while, but you must have cheese or peanut butter, an egg or another protein with the toast.

Plan 1: Food selections

Breakfast options:

Essential protein part of the meal

Eggs cooked any way

Lean bacon, ham, breakfast steak or sausage

Cheese (on toast)—grilled, or soft cheese (ricotta or soft goats cheese) spread thickly on sourdough bread, grilled haloumi

Baked beans (on toast if preferred)

Toast or bread with peanut or other nut butter

Muesli, rolled oats or wholegrain breakfast cereal with high protein milk or with added nuts, LSA* mix added for protein (*LSA mix is a blend of linseeds, sunflower seeds and ground almonds. It's high in protein and good fats as well as fibre.)

Nuts of any variety

Tofu or other soy product or meat alternative

Fuel and antioxidant options to accompany protein

Tomatoes, mushrooms, spinach, any vegetables, herbs and greens

Fruit or dried fruits

Add as many different types and colours of fruits, vegetables, herbs and spices as you can.

Main meal options

Essential protein

Meat of any sort, offal, eggs, cheese, fish, tofu, lentils or other pulses, nuts, quorn and similar

Rice when combined with nuts, pulses or soy products.

Additions

As many vegetables, herbs, spices, fruits as you can fit on your plate—choose a rainbow of colours at every opportunity and aim for the least processed options you can access

Add grain foods—bread, rice, pasta.

Snacks

Snacks are not essential in this plan but if you are active

and not losing weight then include them as you wish. If you need to avoid gaining weight then don't include snacks. Choose mostly natural foods rather than packaged extruded snacks, that includes all sorts of crispy snack foods that look nothing like their original food.

Higher protein options

Yoghurt, egg custard or similar dairy snacks—unsweetened or minimally sweetened ideally and varieties that are NOT low fat usually have fewer thickeners and similar additives

Cheese and carrot or other vegetable sticks

Nuts (or nuts and dried fruit)

Fruit with cheese

Sliced meats

Smoked fish or small cans of tuna/salmon etc.

Antioxidant options

Fruit or dried fruit, fruit juice or fruit and vegetable juice

Biscuits, cakes, etc. that incorporate fruit or vegetables and wholegrains

Fruit toast.

PLAN 2: FOR THOSE WHO HAVE RECENTLY AND UNINTENTIONALLY LOST WEIGHT BUT STILL HAVE A GOOD APPETITE

This plan is designed to give you extra kilojoules as well as the protein and other nutrients you need.

You no longer need to choose low fat foods, so buy full cream milk, yoghurt and dairy foods (it's only three to four percent fat), only trim thick layers of fat from your meat, and choose butter or a quality margarine. Keep milk powder or a high protein supplement in the pantry to make high protein milk, yoghurt, soups, etc.

You should either eat three good meals a day or three smaller meals with snacks in between. You need to try to keep your weight stable, and if you can regain what you've lost that's a bonus. Weigh yourself only once a week, or once every four days at the most, to see how you're going. If you continue to lose weight move to Plan 3, at least for a while.

If you are feeling unwell or not up to eating full meals, or if you don't fancy standard meals, you can choose to eat desserts or have soups or smoothies instead as long as they are high in protein. You can have six to eight good snacks a day instead of meals. It doesn't matter which choice you make as long as they give you what you need.

Plan 2: Food selections

Breakfast options:

Cereal or porridge with high protein milk (recipe for high

protein milk later in this section)

Eggs cooked any way you like them with toast and bacon or other accompaniment. Spread your toast thickly with butter or an alternative spread. If you scramble your eggs use the recipe for high-energy scrambled eggs and add cheese.

Fruit smoothie or milkshake made from high protein drinks (see recipe list)

Bacon, ham, other meat or vegetarian alternative with any accompaniment

Baked beans or similar on toast

Cheese on toast—use thick cheese slices on wholegrain or wholemeal bread with tomato or other herbs or vegetables as desired, or have ricotta or a similar soft cheese

Fruit with high protein yoghurt (see recipe list)

Rice or noodle dish with meat, cheese or nuts added.

Main meals

Meat, fish, seafood, chicken, egg or other animal protein

Vegetarian protein food (pulses, soybeans or soy based product, nuts, seeds) WITH any vegetable, salad or fruit accompaniment and rice or grain food

Pasta, rice or bread may be added to any choice.

If you are struggling to eat adequate meals, boost what's in the meals you can eat: sprinkle a little cheese or chopped ham slices over vegetables or add cheese or nuts to a salad, melt butter over hot vegetables, add cheese sauce to dishes, add high energy gravy to meats (see recipe list).

You can use high protein drinks either between meals or as alternatives to meals if you need to. Choose a commercial supplement or make one from the recipes at the end of this chapter.

Add a dessert

If you have had a good protein food in your main meal then dessert can be anything you fancy. However, if you were not able to eat a good main meal then dessert needs to supply your protein. Choose a high protein dessert from the recipe section.

Snacks

Snacks are useful in this plan if you are not able to eat well at each meal and they are especially important if you are still struggling to keep your weight up. Many of the suggestions in Plan 3 are useful if you have lost weight but are not essential if your weight has stabilised. Whenever possible use snacks to boost your antioxidant intake.

PLAN 3: FOR THOSE WHO HAVE LOST WEIGHT AND ARE STRUGGLING WITH A REDUCED APPETITE

This plan is not 'normal eating'. It's an emergency rehabilitation plan to avoid further weight loss and to halt your rapid loss of independence. If you have become frail and continue to struggle to eat it is perfectly suitable to eat this way for the rest of your life if necessary.

It doesn't matter if you don't eat regular meals any more, or have desserts all day, or even eat the same food at every meal—as long as you get the protein, kilojoules and other nutrients you need.

I haven't divided this list into meals because you can choose any food from the suggestions. Start with six to eight small portions if you can manage it. Weigh yourself about every four days, or once a week. Try to eat every two to three hours. Have small amounts at first, even a spoonful at a time, until you can handle more.

The foods in Plan 3 are all high in kilojoules but you're not likely to gain enough weight for it to be a problem. When your weight stabilises you can move onto Plan 2.

You will need to stock your pantry or fridge with items from the shopping list.

PLAN 3: SHOPPING LIST

High protein supplement powders: there are many varieties on the market. Check with your pharmacist and pharmacy outlets first because the supermarket brands generally don't contain the same range of nutrients.

There are a number of products available in Australian: Enprocal powder (Trisco Foods), Enrich Plus (Enrich Foods NZ), Sustagen (Nestle), Ensure (Abbott) and Advital (Flavour Creations) are some options in Australia. Some are now available unflavoured as well as in the better known vanilla and chocolate flavours. Ensure is lactose free, Enrich Plus is low lactose.

There is also a number of vegan and vegetarian powders available based on soy, hemp, peas or other plant foods, mostly from health food stores, online or from pharmacies.

There is *no reason* to choose artificially sweetened products, in fact the sugar added provides an energy bonus that is very important for people needing this eating plan. Some of these products are unflavoured, but for those that are avoid the artificially sweetened ones, no matter how 'natural' those sweeteners profess to be (you don't need stevia or other low kJ sweeteners).

Whey-based powders: whey is a by-product of cheese production and has been shown to be especially good at improving muscle function in older people. Whey is quite costly, especially the whey protein isolate, which is the most concentrated, but it has shown good results for some older people.

Soy protein isolate is a similar product suitable for vegans.

Body-building powders: these are similar to the powders above and are sold in gyms and health food stores, but it's best to check with your doctor or dietitian first to be sure they are okay for you. Many of these will be artificially sweetened to appeal to the younger market, so look for the unsweetened varieties if they exist and add your own flavours.

Whole or skim milk powders: these can be substituted for the protein milk powders (see above), as their protein content is similar. They cost less but don't contain the range of micronutrients that the more popular commercial supplements do. Full cream milk powder is not as high in protein as skim milk powder but has extra calories and imparts a richer flavour. Either is suitable.

Cheese: cheddar or soft. Ready sliced, cubed or grated cheese, cheeses of any variety, packaged wedges, small portions or cheese sticks (often used for kids' school lunches) are useful to have on hand.

Sliced or barbecued meats: store these in the fridge immediately and throw out any chicken not used after 48 hours.

Ready-to-heat frozen meals: suggestions include party pies, sausage rolls, samosas, chicken drumettes or nuggets, mini quiches, fish cocktails and fish pieces, fish in sauce.

Ready-made meals: try to avoid low fat and 'diet' varieties (and if you buy these, add grated cheese, cream, butter or high protein gravy during reheating to boost their kilojoules).

Pies and quiches

Gravy powder or ready-made gravy and sauces

Yoghurt: preferably NOT low fat. You need to look for those made using full cream milk. Many of the gourmet yoghurts are not low fat, nor are most Greek-style yoghurts.

Other dairy desserts: avoid low fat if possible, but you can always add custard, mousse, crème caramel and cream at home.

Cream: fresh, or buy UHT cream to store in the pantry.

Pate: those made from chicken liver, meat or smoked fish.

Mini ice creams and small tubs: the best are gourmet ice creams that are usually higher in fat, but any will do.

Canned or microwaveable dessert puddings

Soup of any variety including cup-of-soups: prepare with milk powder or neutral flavoured high protein supplement powder to boost their nutrition.

Small cans of fish or meat (chicken is now also widely available)

Baked beans are higher in protein than canned spaghetti.

PLAN 3: MEAL OR SNACK OPTIONS

Choose at least six to eight of these per day:

Commercial drink supplement made to directions

Milkshake or smoothie (see recipe list)

High protein fruit, vegetable juice(see recipe list)

Fruit and vegetable smoothie

Iced coffee with or without sweetening (see recipe list)

High protein yoghurt or custard with a heaped dessertspoon of high protein supplement powder (neutral flavour or vanilla) or milk powder

Fruit with high protein yoghurt

Tuna, salmon or any sort of meat

Small cans of baked beans

Cup-of-soups (or pre-made with one or two heaped dessertspoons of soup) high protein supplement (neutral) or milk powder added

Any of your frozen snack foods reheated

Scrambled egg or boiled. A hard boiled egg with mayonnaise is egg another good option

Egg, cheese or meat sandwich, with a salad preferably

Cheese with crackers or sticks of celery, carrot or apple

Pâté and crackers or toast

Peanut butter on toast

Cheese or baked beans on toast

Ice cream with a heaped spoonful of a flavoured high protein supplement powder (vanilla or chocolate) or sprinkled with chocolate drink powder (Milo, Ovaltine, Akta-Vite)

Handful of nuts or nuts and dried fruit

A couple of slices of cold meat or a piece of cold barbecued chicken

A big spoonful of peanut butter right from the jar!

Breakfast cereal or porridge sprinkled with a heaped spoonful of a vanilla or other flavoured high protein supplement powder

Commercial ready-made meals—if they are diet or low fat meals, add cheese for extra protein and cream for calories

Any vegetable or meat with cheese or mornay sauce

A small can of tuna, salmon or chicken

Commercial snack bars based on nuts or marketed as high protein are good emergency options but many are low fat and sugar free so they're not always ideal.

Sandwich tips

There is no need to avoid butter or margarine. You may put a generous spread on your bread.

In place of butter or margarine, or even in addition, use cream cheese or cheese spread to boost the protein content of your sandwich.

If a whole sandwich is too much, just have one slice of bread but fill it well.

If you are having cold meat, have at least two slices.

Add sliced or grated cheese to as many sandwiches as you can. Salad or tomato is great but the cheese will add protein and calcium too.

Peanut butter or other nut butters are great protein foods for sandwiches.

If you want a sweet sandwich then have one—jam or honey is great—but spread the bread with cream cheese rather than butter to boost the protein and calcium content of your meal.

As an indulgence, spread your bread with butter, then sprinkle a spoonful of Milo or similar powdered drink on your sandwich.

It is possible to turn weight loss around

You can avoid further decline, and also regain some of what has been lost, but it will take a concerted effort. You will have to ignore any mistaken appetite cues to achieve an appreciable return to health and continued independence. You will also have to include an exercise program that you can safely manage. There are many free or very low cost options available in the community.

FOODWORKS

PART 3

Some Recipes and Meal Suggestions

*M*any of these use high protein supplements including milk powder. Most alternatives (soy, hemp, pea) will do the same job, though the flavour may be a bit altered. Check **figure 18** to get an idea of how much to use to get the protein needed.

HIGH PROTEIN COLD DRINKS

High protein milk

1 litre (2 pints) full cream milk (just remove enough from a carton to add the powder)

1 cup skim milk powder, full cream milk powder or unflavoured protein supplement powder.

Sprinkle the powder over milk and mix. Store in the fridge as you would regular milk.

It's best to get a lidded jug that will hold more than a litre then mix the high protein milk and keep it in the fridge. Alternatively, mix the high protein milk and return it to the carton. Use this for all drinks and recipes.

High protein milkshake

Makes 1 serve

200ml (7oz) full cream milk

2 tablespoons high protein supplement powder

Flavouring to taste

Blend and keep any leftover in the fridge for no more than 24 hours.

High protein fruit smoothie

200ml (7oz) full cream milk

2 tablespoons high protein supplement powder

1 piece of fruit or half a cup of berries (peeled or seeded as necessary)

Sugar or honey to taste if required

Blend in a food processor until fruit is thoroughly combined. Store any leftover in the fridge for no more than 24 hours.

High protein green boost drink

200ml (7oz) juice or milk

Bunched handful of kale or similar leafy green vegetable

Handful of raw nuts such as almonds

2 tablespoons of unflavoured high protein supplement powder

Sugar or honey to taste

Blend in a food processor until thoroughly mixed. Store any leftover in the fridge for no more than 24 hours.

HIGH PROTEIN HOT DRINKS

Note: most high protein supplements will curdle if boiled or made with boiling water, so always add powders after heating the other ingredients.

High protein coffee, tea or chai

You can use high protein milk to make these, but also add 1 tablespoon of powdered supplement or milk powder to your drink. If you don't use the high protein milk, add 2 tablespoons powder.

Milo, Horlicks, Ovaltine or similar: These powders are all quite good protein sources—ideally make them with high protein milk.

Cup of soup or home-made soup: Make according to your recipe or packet directions then cool slightly and add 2 tablespoons of skim milk powder or neutral flavour protein supplement per person.

OTHER HIGH PROTEIN RECIPES

High protein breakfast options

Breakfast cereal or

porridge   Use high protein milk on your cereal or sprinkle 2 tablespoons vanilla flavoured supplement powder on top of your cereal or porridge. Add 2 tablespoons of extra nuts – chopped or ground - or LSA mix.

When making porridge, slightly cool the porridge then add 2 tablespoons of skim milk powder or unflavoured protein supplement per person. You can also add ground nuts or LSA mix to porridge during cooking: use about 2 tablespoons per half cup of raw oats to boost protein and good oils.

Eggs: Add 1 tablespoon of skim milk powder to your mix for scrambled eggs before they are cooked, and melt a handful of grated cheese in at the end. Sprinkle over plenty of chopped herbs for extra antioxidants. Add ham, bacon or smoked salmon if desired.

Yoghurt: Add nuts and fruit to Greek yoghurt: to 1 cup yoghurt, add 1 handful of nuts of any sort, plus 4 tablespoons of LSA mix and as many berries or other fruit as you wish.

Other options: Grilled haloumi (about the size of a pack of cards) with avocado and/or salad greens.

High protein gravy

Make up gravy mix with hot or boiling water according to directions, cool slightly. Add 2 tablespoons of skim milk powder or neutral flavour protein supplement per person.

For use in a casserole, add 2 tablespoons of skim milk powder or neutral flavour protein supplement per person to hot (but not boiling) liquid stock. Add this to a pre-cooked casserole just before serving.

High protein custard or dairy dessert

Make custard according to directions then remove from heat, cool a little and stir in 2 tablespoons of skim milk powder or unflavoured protein supplement per person.

High protein jelly

This will make an opaque dessert rather than clear jelly, but the taste is similar and less milky than custard. Make jelly according to directions then cool slightly and add 2 tablespoons of skim milk powder or neutral flavour protein supplement per person. Whisk until dissolved and allow to set as usual.

High protein biscuits, cake or pikelets

Make according to your usual recipe adding 2 tablespoons of skim milk powder or unflavoured protein supplement per person to the flour before mixing it in. Cook as usual.

ADDITIONAL RECIPE IDEAS

Any of the (unflavoured) supplement powders or milk powder can be added to mashed potato. Use 2 tablespoons per person as a guide.

Ground nuts or seeds (including LSA mix—a blend of linseed or flax seeds, sunflower seeds and almonds) make great protein additions as well as high-fibre additives in drinks and even baked goods and casseroles. Add about 2 tablespoons per person.

Foodworks:

Take home from this section:

> › Eat real food—only supplement vitamins and minerals if you have a diagnosed deficiency

> › If your appetite is low, try getting fluid from liquids that also contain nutrients

> › Choose an eating plan that suits your needs

> › Sometimes you just need to snack until you can get back to full meals.

FURTHER READING
AND RESOURCES

Places to go to learn more and extra reading for those who are keen to know a bit more

BODYWORKS

Places to go to learn more:

About exercise:

> www.activeageingaustralia.com.au produces an excellent home exercising book and DVD to give you additional guidance on exercises and intensities

> COTA (Council On The Ageing) runs a fabulous low-cost program called Strength For Life, which can be accessed through your state COTA branch in Australia. Find programs being run locally by typing COTA Strength For Life into your search engine and choosing your state.

> Said, C, Sherrington, C, Hill, K, Callisaya, M, Batchelor, F, Hill, AM, Dawson, R, Mackintosh, S & Fu, S August 2020, Australian Physiotherapy Association, <https://www.safeexerciseathome.org.au>

> Look for Accredited Exercise Physiologists in your local area. These allied health practitioners are able to

design exercises to align with your individual needs.

> Seguin, RA, Epping, JN, Buchner, DM, Bloch, R & Nelson, ME 2002, *Growing Stronger: Strength Training for Older Adults,* Tufts University, <https://www.cdc.gov/physicalactivity/downloads/growing-stronger.pdf>

About food and some reading for people who can cope with a bit of scientific jargon:

> My colleague Catherine Saxelby's Food and Nutrition Companion book is an excellent resource for anyone wanting more information on all manner of things food:

Saxelby, C 2018, *Complete Food And Nutrition Companion,* Hardie Grant, Melbourne.

> Some advice on protein supplementation for athletes from Sports Dietitians Australia:

Sports Dietitians Australia, 2014, *Protein Supplementation,* <https://www.sportsdietitians.com.au/factsheets/supplements/protein-supplementation>

> van Vliet, S, Burd, NA & van Loon, LJC 2015, 'The Skeletal Muscle Anabolic Response to Plant- versus Animal-Based Protein Consumption', *The Journal of Nutrition*, vol. 145(9), pp. 1981-1991, <https://academic.oup.com/jn/article/145/9/1981/4585688>

> Volpi, E, Campbell, W, Dwyer, J, Johnson, M, Jensen, G, Morley, J & Wolfe, R 2012, 'Is the Optimal Level of Protein Intake for Older Adults Greater Than the Recommended Dietary Allowance?' *The Journals of Gerontology Series A: Biological Sciences and Medical Sciences,* vol. 68(6), pp. 677-681.

BRAINWORKS

Places to go to learn more:

> Queensland Brain Institute has a lot of information: The Queensland Brain Institute, 2020, University of Queensland, <https://qbi.uq.edu.au/brain-basics>

> The University of Tasmania runs a free online program, called MOOC (multi online open course) on Understanding Dementia:
> Wicking Dementia Research and Education Centre 2020, *Understanding Dementia MOOC,* University of Tasmania, <https://www.utas.edu.au/wicking/understanding-dementia>

A bit of extra reading for those who can cope with a bit of scientific jargon:

> More on glia: Neuro Transmissions, 2016, *Glorious Glia: What Are Astrocytes?* <https://alieastrocyte.wordpress.com/2016/08/28/glorious-glia-what-are-astrocytes/>

> More on the blood-brain-barrier: Rhea, EM & Banks WA 2019, 'Role of the the Blood-Brain Barrier in Central Nervous System Insulin Resistance, *Front, Neurosci*, vol. 13:521 <https://www.frontiersin.org/articles/10.3389/fnins.2019.00521/full>

> Some information on the supplement *Souvenaid*: Alzheimer's Society 2020, *Souvenaid: I'm worried about my memory – should I buy this drink?* <https://www.alzheimers.org.uk/blog/souvenaid-im-worried-about-my-memory-should-i-buy-drink>

> And for those who relish a good delve into scientific

research:

> Arnold, S, Arvanitakis, Z, Macauley-Rambach, S, Koenig, A, Wang, H, Ahima, R, Craft, S, Gandy, S, Buettner, C, Stoeckel, L, Holtzman, D & Nathan, D 2018, 'Brain insulin resistance in type 2 diabetes and Alzheimer disease: concepts and conundrums', *Nature Reviews Neurology*, vol. 14(3), pp. 168-181.

> Choudhry, H & Nasrullah, M 2018, 'Iodine consumption and cognitive performance: Confirmation of adequate consumption', *Food Science & Nutrition*, vol. 6(6), pp. 1341-1351.

> Le Chatelier, E, Nielsen T, Qin, J, et al. 2013, 'Richness of human gut microbiome correlates with metabolic markers', *Nature*, vol. 500(7464), pp. 541-546.

> Nowotny, K, Shruter, D, Schreiner, M & Grune, T 2018, 'Dietary advanced glycation end products and their relevance for human health', *Ageing Research Reviews*, Vol 47, pp. 55-66

> Oriach, CR, Robertson, RC, Stanton, C, Cryan, JF & Dinan, TG 2016, 'Food for thought: The role of nutrition in the microbiota-gut–brain axis', *Clinical Nutrition Experimental*, April 6, pp. 25-38.

> Uribarri, J, Woodruff, S, Goodman, S, Cai, W, Chen, X, Young, A, Striker, GE & Vlassara, H 2010, 'Advanced glycation end products in foods and a practical guide to their reduction in the diet', *J Am Diet Assoc*, vol. 110(6), pp. 911-916

HEALTHWORKS

Places to go to learn more:

To find a dietitian:

> Dietitians Australia 2020, Dietitians Association of Australia, <https://dietitiansaustralia.org.au>

To find a speech pathologist:

> Speech Pathology Australia 2016, <https://www.speechpathologyaustrali.org.au>

Some oral health information for older adults that might be useful:

> The Australian Dental Association has some good general information on Oral Health at Later Age here: https://www.ada.org.au/Your-Dental-Health/Older-Adults-65

And some extra reading for those who can cope with a bit more scientific jargon:

> Agarwal, E, Ferguson, M, Banks, M, Vivanti, A, Batterham, M, Bauer, J, Capra, S & Isenring, E 2019, 'Malnutrition, poor food intake, and adverse healthcare outcomes in non-critically ill obese acute care hospital patients', *Clinical Nutrition*, vol. 38 (2), pp. 759-766.

> Coll, PP, Lindsay, A, Meng, J, Gopalakrishna, A, Raghavendra, S, Bysani, P & O'Brien, D 2020, 'The Prevention of Infections in Older Adults: Oral Health', *J Am Geriatr Soc*, vol. 68, pp. 411-416.

> Pujia, A, Gazzaruso, C, Ferro, Y, Mazza, E, Maurotti, S, Russo, C & Montalcini, T 2016, 'Individuals with metabolically healthy overweight/obesity have higher fat utilization than metabolically unhealthy individuals', *Nutrients*, vol. 8(1).

> Sinclair, A, Dunning, T & Rodriguez-Mañas, L 2015, 'Diabetes in older people: New insights and remaining challenges', *The Lancet Diabetes and Endocrinology*, vol. 3(4), pp. 275-285.

FOODWORKS

Places to go to learn more:

Some good higher protein recipe and food resources:

> Meat and Livestock Australia 2015, <https://www.mlahealthymeals.com.au/resources/#>

> Nuts for Life 2020, https://www.nutsforlife.com.au/recipes

> Dairy Australia, https://www.dairy.com.au/recipes

A place to access nutritional supplements and texture modified food products

BrightSky is a company distributing a wide range of products including commercial nutrition supplementary and texture modified foods and drinks in Australia. Search their online shop at: https://www.brightsky.com.au/

More on Meniere's disease, salt and potassium:

> Henderson, K 2018, *Meniere's Disease: Potassium and Salt. The Importance of Keeping a Healthy Balance*, <https://www.menieres-disease.ca/salt-and-potassium

More info on diet for those with thyroid problems:

> British Thyroid Foundation 2019, <https://www.btf-thyroid.org/thyroid-and-diet-factsheet>

More info on IBS and FODMAPs

> International Foundation for Gastrointestinal Disorders 2016, *What is IBS?*, https://www.aboutibs.org/what-is-ibs.html

> Monash University 2019, The Low FODMAP Diet, https://www.monashfodmap.com

Psychological treatment for IBS

> Anxiety Treatment Australia 2020, <https://www.anxietyaustralia.com.au/resources/irritable-bowel-syndrome-ibs-stress-and-anxiety/>

A bit of extra reading for those who relish a good delve into scientific research:

> Li, K, Wang, XF, Li, DY, Chen, YC, Zhao, LJ, Liu, XG, Guo, YF, Shen, J, Xu, L, Deng, J, Zhou, R & Deng, HW 2018, 'The good, the bad, and the ugly of calcium supplementation: a review of calcium intake on human health', *Clin Interv Aging*, Vol.13, pp. 2443-2452.

> Marian, M & Sacks, G 2009, 'Micronutrients and older

adults', *Nutrition in Clinical Practice: official publication of the American Society for Parenteral and Enteral Nutrition,* vol. 24(2), pp. 179-95.

› Sandoval-Insausti, H, Blanco-Rojo, R, Graciani, A, Lopez-Garcia, E, Moreno-Franco, B, Laclaustra, M, Donat-Vargas, C, Ordovas, JM, Rodriguez-Artalejo, F & Guallar-Castillon, P 2020, 'Ultra-processed Food Consumption and Incident Frailty: A Prospective Cohort Study of Older Adults', *The Journals of Gerontology*, Vol. 75 (6), pp. 1126–1133.

Some extra reading on protein quality and muscle throughout life:

› Burd, NA, McKenna, CF, Salvador, AF, Paulussen, KJM & Moore, DR 2019, 'Dietary Protein Quantity, Quality, and Exercise are Key to Healthy Living: A Muscle-Centric Perspective Across the Lifespan', *Front, Neurosci*, June,

<https://www.frontiersin.org/articles/10.3389/fnut.2019.00083/full>

INDEX

A

AGEs (advanced glycation end
products), 80 - 83

ALA, 97

Alzheimer's disease, 136 - 137

accumulation of iron and ,99

and folate, 256

and glucose supply, 76

and homocysteine levels, 254

and Omega 3 fats, 76

and special food supplements
133

and vitamin B6, 254

amino acids, 23, 93, 211, 239

antioxidant vitamins, 101

antioxidants, 82, 101-2, 113, 121-
5, 133, 146, 214-6, 242-3

appetite:

effect of medication on, 187-
190

poor or reduced, 88, 120, 179-
185

arginine, 211

aspiration, 201-2

aspirin, low dose, 258

astrocytes, 72, 86-7

B

B vitamins – see under vitamins

bacteria, see microbiome, gut microbiome

basal metabolic rate (BMR), 141

BDNF, 69, 71, 116, 121, 129

Bed rest, 28, 62

Beta (or β) Amyloid, 77, 79-80, 97,
100

bisphosphonates, 58-9

blood brain barrier, 93, 112, 124,

and obesity, 37

blood flow and brain function, 109-
110

dehydration and, 87

blood glucose

controlling, 84, 162-4, 170-4

high, 79, 80,

low, 79-80,

blood pressure

effect on the brain, 111

low - postural hypotension, 111

blood vessels

blood pressure and, 111

diabetes and, 73, 79-80,

and brain, 109, 111

Body Mass Index (BMI), 42, 44-5,

bowel

www.ingramcontent.com/pod-product-compliance
Lightning Source LLC
Chambersburg PA
CBHW060027030426
42334CB00019B/2216